PREFACE

The four-volume text *Diagnosis of Diseases of the Chest,* third edition, was based on two premises: (1) that one of the early steps in the diagnosis of diseases of the chest should be an assessment of the pattern of changes revealed on a chest roentgenogram, and (2) that correlation of these findings with the clinical history and with abnormalities revealed by physical examination, laboratory investigation, pulmonary function testing, and special investigations will yield a positive diagnosis in the majority of cases. If this proposition is accepted, clearly it is necessary to evaluate the chest roentgenogram on the basis of pattern recognition in which individual patterns can be related to pathogenesis and thence to etiology. To describe a roentgenographic shadow as an "infiltrate" says no more than that the lung is the site of an opacity; to describe the *pattern* that the opacity possesses—homogeneous or inhomogeneous, segmental or nonsegmental, air-space or interstitial—constitutes an attempt to assess the *mechanism* by which the disease developed and thus to suggest its cause.

With these sequences in mind, we compiled 17 tables of differential diagnosis that list all the basic roentgenographic patterns of chest disease, each table providing a nosologic approach to the differential diagnosis of disease of that pattern. Within the tables, the classification of disease is on an etiologic basis, categories being arranged in the same order as the chapters in the book—e.g., developmental, infectious, immunologic, neoplastic, and so on. Each table includes *all* common diseases and the *majority* of uncommon diseases which produce that particular pattern. The search for rare conditions in order to achieve completeness has not been exhaustive, since we feared that the tables would become too cumbersome to be of practical use. In addition, our desire to reduce length to practical proportions was hindered by the necessity for repetition: considerable overlap of patterns was inevitable, necessitating the inclusion of the same diseases in several tables.

These 17 tables of differential diagnosis are included in the four-volume set as an Appendix in Volume IV, a book of almost 750 pages. Since a book of such bulk is hardly conducive to being carried around for repeated consultation, it was decided to produce a small "pocket" edition that included only the tables of differential diagnosis. This little book is intended for use by radiology and pulmonology residents, respiratory therapists, and physicians and surgeons whose practice involves the interpretation of chest roentgenograms and the differential diagnosis of abnormalities revealed thereon.

These tables of differential diagnosis are designed to be used in the following manner. First, refer to the descriptions of the characteristics of each specific pattern that precede the tables. When a specific roentgenographic pattern is recognized, the appropriate table is consulted and reviewed. The headings in each table are intended to provide a brief review of the characteristics of each disease that might aid in differentiating it from others that cause the same pattern. Thus, the most likely diagnostic possibilities are selected. Should additional information be desired concerning a specific disease entity, the four-volume text can be referred to on the page referenced in the righthand column of the tables.

ROBERT G. FRASER, M.D.
J.A. PETER PARÉ, M.D.
P.D. PARÉ, M.D.
RICHARD S. FRASER, M.D.

CONTENTS

TABLE 1

**Homogeneous Opacities Without Recognizable
Segmental Distribution**

This pattern is epitomized by acute airspace pneumonia caused by *Streptococcus pneumoniae*. Typically the inflammation begins in the subpleural parenchyma and spreads centrifugally through pores of Kohn; since segmental boundaries do not impede such spread, consolidation tends to be nonsegmental. An air bronchogram is almost invariable and should not be misinterpreted as evidence of inhomogeneity. If the distribution of the disease is roughly segmental (for example, when acute airspace pneumonia fills a whole lobe), the presence of an air bronchogram should take precedence over apparent segmental distribution in suggesting the pathogenesis and therefore the etiology of the disease.

The nonsegmental character of parenchymal consolidation relates largely to its pathogenesis. For example, the volume of lung affected by acute irradiation pneumonitis corresponds roughly to the area irradiated, with little tendency to segmental or lobar distribution.

1

TABLE 1
Homogeneous Opacities Without Recognizable Segmental Distribution

Etiology	Loss of Volume	Anatomic Distribution	Additional Findings	Comments
DEVELOPMENTAL Pulmonary arteriovenous fistula	0	Lower lobe predilection.	Fairly extensive racemose opacity, ill-defined but homogeneous, occupying much of one bronchopulmonary segment (but not truly segmental).	Represents a complex angiomatous mass possessing one or more feeding and draining vessels. (*See* page 752.)
INFECTIOUS **Bacteria** *Streptococcus pneumoniae.*	0 to +	Influence of gravity; therefore dependent portions of upper and lower lobes. Usually unilobar.	Air bronchogram almost invariable; fairly sharply circumscribed margins, even where not abutting against fissure; cavitation rare except with superimposed anaerobic infection.	Confluent airspace consolidation begins in subpleural parenchyma and spreads centrifugally via pores of Kohn; therefore no tendency to segmental involvement. (*See* page 831.)
Klebsiella-Enterobacter-Serratia species.	Tendency to expansion of involved lung, although volume may be normal or even reduced.	Upper lobe predilection; often multilobar.	Cavitation common; air bronchogram almost invariable; pleural effusion may be present.	Differs from pneumococcal pneumonia in propensity to cavitation and tendency to expand involved lung. (*See* page 846.)

2

Mycobacterium tuberculosis (primary).	0 to +	Slightly more frequent in upper lobes; no predilection for either anterior or posterior segments.	Ipsilateral hilar or paratracheal lymph node enlargement almost invariable in children but in only about 50 per cent of adults. Pleural effusion in 10 per cent of affected children (almost always associated with parenchymal disease) and in approximately one third of adults (often as the sole manifestation). Cavitation and miliary spread rare.	(*See* page 891.)
Mycobacterium tuberculosis (postprimary).	0 to +	Upper lobe predilection, predominantly posterior (influence of gravity on endobronchial spread).	Cavitation common. Individual acinar shadows frequently identifiable elsewhere in lungs due to endobronchial spread. Air bronchogram invariable.	Acute tuberculous pneumonia. Infection may transgress interlobar fissures from one lobe to another or occasionally may extend into chest wall and form abscesses (empyema necessitatis). (*See* page 915.)
Francisella tularensis (tularemia).	0	No lobar predilection; may be multilobar.	Hilar lymph node enlargement and pleural effusion common; cavitation rare.	May be extensive involvement of both lungs; oval or spherical homogeneous consolidation. (*See* page 870.)
Legionella pneumophila.	0 to +	Usually unilateral and unilobar when first seen, with tendency to multilobar and bilateral involvement with time. Lower lobe predilection.	Abscess formation uncommon except in immunocompromised patients. Pleural effusion in 35 to 63 per cent of cases.	Consolidation may progress rapidly despite antibiotic therapy. Resolution is often prolonged. (*See* page 861.)
Pseudomonas aeruginosa.	0	Generalized or nonspecific.	Pleural effusion common.	Less common method of presentation than homogeneous segmental consolidation (Table 2). The majority of infections are acquired in hospital. (*See* page 855.)

3

Table continued on following page

Etiology	Loss of Volume	Anatomic Distribution	Additional Findings	Comments
INFECTIOUS *(Continued)*				
Bacteria *(Continued)*				
Pseudomonas pseudomallei.	0	Single or multiple lobes.	———	Homogeneous consolidation due to confluence of multiple areas of airspace consolidation. Involvement may be extensive, resembling pulmonary edema. *(See page 860.)*
Haemophilus influenzae.	0	No lobar predilection.	Effusion common.	Uncommon presentation. *(See page 853.)*
Yersinia pestis (the Black Plague).	0	No lobar predilection.	Pleural effusion in some cases.	May be overwhelming infection, with multilobar involvement and pulmonary edema pattern simulating ARDS. *(See page 850.)*
Anaerobic bacteria.	0	Posterior portion of upper or lower lobes.	Tends to progress to lung abscess.	Acute airspace pneumonia tends to occur when aspirate is of watery consistency. *(See page 895.)*
Escherichia coli.	0	Strong lower lobe anatomic bias, usually multilobar.	Pleural effusion frequent; cavitation uncommon.	Affects chiefly debilitated patients. *(See page 849.)*
Actinomyces israelii (actinomycosis). *Nocardia* species (nocardiosis).	0	Lower lobe predilection, often bilateral.	Cavitation common; pleural effusion and extension into chest wall characteristic (with or without rib destruction). Similarly, may transgress interlobar fissures from one lobe to another.	Roentgenographic patterns of these organisms are indistinguishable. *(See pages 1024 and 1028.)*

Fungi

Blastomyces dermatitidis (blastomycosis).	0	Upper lobe predilection in ratio of 3:2.	Cavitation uncommon (15 per cent); pleural effusion and lymph node enlargement rare, as is chest wall involvement.	Contrast with actinomycosis and nocardiosis in frequency of cavitation, pleural effusion, and chest wall involvement. (*See* page 970.)
Histoplasma capsulatum (histoplasmosis).	0	No predilection.	Hilar lymph node enlargement common; cavitation may occur.	This pneumonic type is considerably less common than inhomogeneous primary histoplasmosis. (*See* page 947.)
Coccidioides immitis (coccidioidomycosis).	0	Lower lobe predilection.	Hilar and paratracheal lymph node enlargement may be present; cavitation common.	(*See* page 958.)
Candida albicans (candidiasis).	0	No predilection.	May cavitate.	Less common presentation than inhomogeneous segmental pattern (*see* Table 4). (*See* page 987.)
Geotrichum candidum (geotrichosis).	0	Upper lobe predilection.	Cavitation common, usually thin-walled.	(*See* page 1018.)
Aspergillus species (invasive aspergillosis).	0	No predilection.	Cavitation uncommon.	Much less common form of disease than fungus ball or mucoid impaction. (*See* page 1007.)
Cryptococcus neoformans (cryptococcosis).	0	Lower lung zones.	Cavitation uncommon, as is node enlargement.	Less common roentgenographic presentation than a discrete mass. (*See* page 977.)

5

Table continued on following page

TABLE 1
Homogeneous Opacities Without Recognizable Segmental Distribution *(Continued)*

Etiology	Loss of Volume	Anatomic Distribution	Additional Findings	Comments
INFECTIOUS *(Continued)*				
Parasites				
Entamoeba histolytica (amebiasis).	0	Right lower lobe almost exclusively.	Right pleural effusion very common. Cavitation occurs in minority of cases.	Organisms enter thorax via diaphragm from liver abscesses. (*See* page 1081.)
Paragonimus westermani (paragonimiasis).	0	No predilection.	Isolated nodular shadows, usually cavitary; may be pleural effusion.	Organisms enter thorax via diaphragm; spread via bronchial tree. (*See* page 1109.)
Ascaris lumbricoides (ascariasis).	0	Multilobar.	———	Löffler-type pattern suggested by fleeting nature of consolidation. (*See* page 1093.)
Strongyloides stercoralis.	0	Multilobar.	———	Löffler-type pattern. (*See* page 1094.)
Ancylostoma duodenale.	0	Multilobar.	———	Löffler-type pattern. (*See* page 1097.)
Pneumocystis carinii.	0	Generalized.	Pleural effusion very uncommon.	Massive airspace consolidation represents the terminal stage of pulmonary disease. (*See* page 1085.)
IMMUNOLOGIC				
Löffler's syndrome.	0	Peripherally situated without lobar predilection.	Foci of consolidation may be single or multiple, generally ill-defined and transitory or migratory in character. Cavitation, pleural effusion, lymph node enlargement, and cardiomegaly do not occur. Eosinophilia invariable.	Main differential diagnosis is allergic bronchopulmonary aspergillosis. (*See* page 1291.)

Chronic eosinophilic pneumonia.	0	Peripheral lung zones without lobar predilection.	Blood eosinophilia common but not invariable.	In contrast to Löffler's syndrome, lesions tend to remain unchanged for days or weeks. Response to corticosteroid therapy characteristically dramatic. (*See* page 1292.)
Polyarteritis nodosa (PAN).	0	Peripheral lung zones, without lobar predilection.	Consolidation tends to be patchy and fleeting in nature and thus indistinguishable from Löffler's syndrome.	Whether pulmonary disease is caused by PAN *per se* is controversial; the majority of roentgenographic abnormalities are probably attributable to chronic renal disease, hypertension, or cardiac decompensation. (*See* page 1253.)

NEOPLASTIC

Hodgkin's disease.	0	No predilection.	Almost invariably associated with hilar or mediastinal lymph node enlargement. Pleural effusion in 30 per cent of cases. Air bronchogram almost invariable.	Individual lesions may coalesce to form larger areas of homogeneous consolidation. (*See* page 1507.)
Non-Hodgkin's lymphoma.	0	No predilection.	Often without associated hilar and mediastinal node enlargement. Pleural effusion in one third. Air bronchogram invariable.	(*See* page 1535.)
Bronchiolo-alveolar carcinoma.	0	No predilection.	Air bronchogram invariable.	Malignant cells may be found in sputum, which is usually mucoid and sometimes copious. (*See* page 1414.)

Table continued on following page

TABLE 1
Homogeneous Opacities Without Recognizable Segmental Distribution *(Continued)*

Etiology	Loss of Volume	Anatomic Distribution	Additional Findings	Comments
TRAUMATIC				
Pulmonary parenchymal contusion.	0 to +	Usually in lung directly deep to area traumatized, although it may develop as well or even predominantly on the side opposite from the trauma due to contracoup effect. No conformity to lobes or segments.	Roentgenographic changes develop soon after trauma, almost invariably within six hours. Increase in size and loss of definition of vascular markings extending out from the hila indicate hemorrhage and edema in the major interstitial space.	The most common pulmonary complication of blunt chest trauma. The roentgenographic pattern varies from irregular patchy areas of airspace consolidation to diffuse and extensive homogeneous consolidation. Consolidation results from exudation of edema fluid and blood into the parenchyma of the lung in both its airspace and interstitial components. *(See* page 2481.)
Acute irradiation pneumonitis.	+ + to + + + +	The volume of lung affected generally but not always corresponds to the area irradiated; no tendency to segmental or lobar distribution.	Despite severe loss of volume, segmental bronchi tend to be unaffected so that an air bronchogram is almost invariable. Roentgenographically demonstrable pleural effusion is very uncommon although there may be fairly extensive thickening of the pleura.	The reaction of the lung to irradiation is affected by a number of variables including the dosage of radiation administered, the time over which it is given, the site to which the radiation is directed, and the condition of the lung prior to irradiation. *(See* page 2551.)

| Lung torsion. | 0 to + | A whole lobe or lung. | Torsion occurs through 180 degrees so that the base of the lung or lobe comes to lie at the apex of the hemithorax and the apex at the base: the pattern of pulmonary vascular markings is thus altered in a predictable manner. | If torsion is not relieved, vascular supply is compromised and the lung becomes opaque owing to exudation of blood into the airspaces and interstitial tissues. (*See* page 2494.) |

TABLE 2

Homogeneous Opacities of Recognizable Segmental Distribution

The pattern is caused most often by endobronchial obstructing lesions — segmental atelectasis with or without obstructive pneumonitis. Since the pathogenesis involves bronchial obstruction, the resultant shadow necessarily is of specific bronchopulmonary segmental distribution. An air bronchogram should be absent except when the atelectasis is "adhesive" or "nonobstructive" in type or when therapy has relieved the obstruction, thereby permitting the entry of air into the involved segmental bronchi.

Acute confluent bronchopneumonia, commonly of staphylococcal etiology, also produces this pattern. The pathogenesis of bronchopneumonia implies a segmental distribution; the virulence of the infection results in confluence of consolidation and consequent homogeneity. As in obstructive pneumonitis, an air bronchogram seldom is present.

TABLE 2
Homogeneous Opacities of Recognizable Segmental Distribution

Etiology	Loss of Volume	Anatomic Distribution	Additional Findings	Comments
DEVELOPMENTAL Pulmonary arteriovenous fistula	+ to + + + +	Predilection for lower lobes.	The feeding artery and draining vein may be partly or completely obscured by the shadow of the collapsed segment.	Bronchial compression with resultant atelectasis or obstructive pneumonitis is a rare complication. (*See* page 752.)
INFECTIOUS **Bacteria** *Staphylococcus aureus.*	0 to + +	No lobar predilection.	Abscess formation common; pleural effusion (empyema) common, particularly in children, with or without bronchopleural fistula (pyopneumothorax).	This is confluent bronchopneumonia; air bronchogram exceptional. Disease is bilateral in over 60 per cent of adults. (*See* page 836.)
Mycobacterium tuberculosis (primary).	0 to + + + +	2:1 predominance of right lung over left; predilection for anterior segment of upper lobe or medial segment of middle lobe.	Associated paratracheal or hilar lymph node enlargement in two thirds of patients.	Atelectasis results either from compression from enlarged lymph nodes or from endobronchial tuberculosis. In adults, tuberculous bronchostenosis tends to show a female sex predominance and a lower lobe predilection. (*See* page 891.)
Streptococcus pneumoniae.	0 to +	Influence of gravity; therefore dependent portions of upper and lower lobes.	Air bronchogram almost invariable; cavitation rare.	True segmental distribution very uncommon, and only when whole lobe involved. (*See* page 828.)

12

Streptococcus pyogenes.	0 to + +	Predominantly lower lobes.	Pleural effusion almost invariable.	As confluent bronchopneumonia, this is a more common method of presentation than inhomogeneous involvement. (*See* page 835.)
Pseudomonas aeruginosa.	0 to + +	Predominantly lower lobes.	Abscess formation with empyema common, with or without bronchopleural fistula (pyopneumothorax).	Confluent bronchopneumonia; a more common method of presentation than homogeneous nonsegmental consolidation. (*See* page 855.)
Bordetella (*Haemophilus*) *pertussis* (whooping cough pneumonia).	+ to + +	Predominantly lower lobes.	"Shaggy heart" sign. Hilar node enlargement in 30 per cent of patients.	Confluent bronchopneumonia, associated with some degree of atelectasis in at least 50 per cent of cases; pneumonia may be caused by secondary invader or by *Bordetella pertussis* itself. (*See* page 869.)
Anaerobic organisms.	0 to + +	Reflects influence of gravity— posterior segments of upper lobes and superior segment of lower lobes.	Abscess formation in the majority of cases. Empyema common.	Results from aspiration of anaerobically infected material in patients with poor oral hygiene. Tends to have a protracted, insidious course. (*See* page 875.)
All other bacteria listed in Table 4.	0 to + +	Predominantly lower lobes.	———	These bacteria characteristically produce an inhomogeneous consolidation, but on occasion the densities may be confluent, thus leading to homogeneous consolidation.

Table continued on following page

TABLE 2

Etiology	Loss of Volume	Anatomic Distribution	Additional Findings	Comments
INFECTIOUS *(Continued)*				
Fungi				
Histoplasma capsulatum.	+ to + + + +	Predilection for right middle lobe.	Enlargement of bronchopulmonary lymph nodes an invariable accompaniment.	Compression from enlarged nodes results in obstructive pneumonitis or atelectasis. Calcification of compressing lymph nodes may be associated with erosion into the bronchial lumen (broncholithiasis.) (*See* page 949.)
Mucorales order (mucormycosis).	0 to +	No predilection.	———	Segmental consolidation may occur either from direct parenchymal invasion of the organism (confluent bronchopneumonia) or from pulmonary infarction secondary to pulmonary arterial invasion. (*See* page 1016.)
Other fungi listed in Tables 1 and 4.	0 to +	Predominantly lower lobes.	———	These fungi characteristically produce an inhomogeneous consolidation (bronchopneumonia), but on occasion the densities may be confluent, thus leading to homogeneous consolidation.

Viruses and Rickettsiae

Coxiella burnetii (Q fever).	0	Predominantly lower lobes.	Pleural effusion is occasionally seen. Hilar lymph node enlargement rare.	Extent of consolidation may range from one segment to a complete lobe. (*See* page 1077.)
All viruses listed in Table 4 (as well as *Mycoplasma*).	0 to + + +	Lower lobe predilection.	Pleural effusion and hilar node enlargement very uncommon.	These organisms characteristically cause inhomogeneous segmental consolidation, but on occasion the densities may be confluent. During the stage of resolution of adenoviral pneumonia, particularly in children, there may occur severe adhesive ("nonobstructive") atelectasis; despite the marked loss of volume, an air bronchogram usually is present.

IMMUNOLOGIC

Hypersensitivity bronchopulmonary aspergillosis and mucoid impaction.	0 to + +	Predilection for upper lobes.	Round, oval, or elliptical masses seen in proximal bronchi. The pulmonary parenchyma distal to the mucous plug may be collapsed or show varying degrees of obstructive pneumonitis but commonly contains air due to collateral air drift from contiguous segments. Lungs are often overinflated as a result of associated spasmodic asthma.	Following disappearance of the mucous plugs, there remains a typical pattern of "proximal" bronchiectasis, which is diagnostic. (*See* page 993.)
Wegener's granulomatosis.	+ to + + +	No predilection.	Single or multiple masses, sometimes with cavitation.	Atelectasis caused by endobronchial involvement. (*See* page 1241.)

15

Table continued on following page

Etiology	Loss of Volume	Anatomic Distribution	Additional Findings	Comments
NEOPLASTIC				
Pulmonary carcinoma.	+ to + + + +	The ratio of right to left lung is 6:4 and a similar ratio exists from upper to lower lobes. The neoplasm arises from the main or lobar bronchi in 20 to 40 per cent of cases and from segmental bronchi in 60 to 80 per cent.	The neoplasm may be identified as a mass distinct from the obstructive pneumonitis. Enlarged lymph nodes may be present in the hilum and elsewhere. Pleural effusion in 10 to 15 per cent of cases.	Oligemia and air trapping distal to bronchial obstruction are uncommon manifestations. (*See* page 1368.)
Carcinoid tumor.	+ to + + + +	Tends to arise from large or segmental bronchi. May occur in any lobe without clear-cut lobar predilection.	Typical findings are those of "obstructive pneumonitis." The tumor may be identified on the plain roentgenograms or by CT. Enlarged lymph nodes occasionally may be identified in the hilum or elsewhere. Osseous metastases rare.	In 75 per cent of cases this is the method of presentation of this neoplasm. (*See* page 1477.)
Tracheobronchial gland neoplasms.	+ to + + + +	Lower lobe predilection.	Tend to arise in central airways.	Comprise less than 0.5 per cent of all pulmonary neoplasms. Several distinct histologic varieties have been described. (*See* page 1497).

16

Tracheobronchial papillomas.	+ to + + + +	No predilection.	Endobronchial papillomas are commonly multiple and are associated with similar lesions in the larynx and trachea. Tomography of the larynx, trachea, and lungs may be diagnostic. Bronchiectasis and abscess formation distal to the endobronchial lesions are frequent. Excavation of the lesions may occur.	(*See* page 1502.)
Neoplasms of muscle. Neoplasms of vascular tissue. Neoplasms of bone and cartilage. Neoplasms of neural tissue. Neoplasms of adipose tissue. Neoplasms of fibrohistiocytic tissue. Neoplasms of mixed mesenchymal appearance. Miscellaneous neoplasms of uncertain histogenesis. Miscellaneous tumors of non-neoplastic or uncertain nature.	+ to + + + +	No definite predilection.	———	Rarely any of these neoplasms may arise from the bronchial wall and obstruct the bronchial lumen leading to obstructive pneumonitis. The more common method of presentation is as a solitary nodule. (*See* pages 1577 to 1608.)

17

Table continued on following page

Etiology	Loss of Volume	Anatomic Distribution	Additional Findings	Comments
NEOPLASTIC *(Continued)*				
Hodgkin's disease.	+ to + + + +	No known predilection.	Hilar and/or mediastinal lymph-node enlargement commonly associated. Other patterns of lung involvement also may be associated, particularly parenchymal consolidation presenting as a homogeneous density possessing no recognizable segmental distribution.	Atelectasis (with or without obstructive pneumonitis) results from bronchial obstruction, almost always due to endobronchial involvement by Hodgkin's tissue; rarely may be caused by compression from enlarged lymph nodes. Absence of air bronchogram of differential value. *(See page 1507.)*
Non-Hodgkin's lymphoma.	+ to + + + +	No known lobar predilection.	Hilar and/or mediastinal lymph node enlargement commonly associated. Other patterns of lung involvement also may be associated, particularly parenchymal consolidation presenting as a homogeneous density possessing no recognizable segmental distribution.	Rarely presents as an endobronchial deposit leading to segmental atelectasis and pneumonitis, and only in the secondary form of the disease. *(See page 1545.)*
THROMBOEMBOLIC				
Thromboembolism with infarction.	0 to + +	Lower lobes, usually posteriorly but often nestled in the costophrenic sinus; less than 10 per cent in upper lobes. May be multiple.	Ipsilateral hemidiaphragm frequently raised; increase in size and abrupt tapering of feeder artery is characteristic; pleural effusion is common. Signs of postcapillary hypertension due to associated cardiac disease may be present.	The size of the infarcted area is generally 3 to 5 cm in diameter but ranges from barely visible to 10 cm in diameter; occasionally shows truncated cone appearance ("Hampton's hump"). *(See page 1724.)*

18

INHALATIONAL

Aspiration of solid foreign bodies.	+ to + + + +	Lower lobes almost exclusively, ratio of right to left being 2:1.	The foreign body is opaque (e.g., a tooth) in approximately 10 per cent of patients.	Segmental collapse or consolidation occurs in only 25 per cent of cases, the remainder being categorized by "obstructive overinflation." (*See* page 2382.)
Lipoid pneumonia. 0 to +		Generally dependent portions of lower and upper lobes (occasionally right middle lobe or lingula).	None.	The characteristic roentgenographic pattern is alveolar consolidation, commonly homogeneous but sometimes associated with isolated acinar shadows, particularly in the early stages of the disease. The segmental nature of the consolidation may be quite precise. (*See* page 2398.)

TRAUMATIC

Bronchial fracture.	+ + to + + + +	One or more lobes or an entire lung.	Pneumothorax, pneumomediastinum, and subcutaneous emphysema. Fractures of the first three ribs frequently associated, particularly in adults (53 per cent of cases).	Atelectasis develops as a result of displacement of fracture ends and is commonly a late development. The occurrence of atelectasis sometime after an accident should strongly suggest the diagnosis (additional confirmatory evidence provided by fractures of one or more of the first three ribs). (*See* page 2485.)
Postoperative adhesive atelectasis.	+ to + + +	Left lower lobe predilection.	The usual findings associated with postoperative thoracotomy — pleural effusion, diaphragmatic elevation, and so forth.	Occurs predominantly following cardiac surgery, particularly with use of extracorporeal circulation. The degree of collapse varies considerably. Since the mechanism of atelectasis operates peripherally, an air bronchogram is invariable. (*See* page 2532.)

19

Table continued on following page

TABLE 2
Homogeneous Opacities of Recognizable Segmental Distribution *(Continued)*

Etiology	Loss of Volume	Anatomic Distribution	Additional Findings	Comments
METABOLIC Bronchopulmonary amyloidosis.	+ to + + +	No predilection.	Sometimes associated with solitary or multiple pulmonary nodules or masses.	Atelectasis or obstructive pneumonitis is caused by intramural masses of amyloid. (*See* page 2578.)
IDIOPATHIC Sarcoidosis.	+ to + + + +	No predilection.	Almost invariably associated with more characteristic changes such as hilar and mediastinal lymph node enlargement and a diffuse reticulonodular pattern.	A rare complication of endobronchial sarcoidosis that may be suspected from other roentgenographic findings and can be confirmed by bronchoscopy and bronchial biopsy. (*See* page 2611.)

TABLE 3

Inhomogeneous Opacities Without Recognizable Segmental Distribution

Postprimary tuberculosis undoubtedly is the most common cause of this pattern — focal areas of parenchymal consolidation separated by zones of air-containing lung. Although tuberculosis commonly is localized to the apical and posterior *regions* of an upper lobe, it seldom is truly segmental; in other words, it does not tend to affect a pyramidal section of lung of which the apex is at the hilum and base at the visceral pleura. It must be emphasized that the presence of cavitation *in itself* should not be interpreted as a cause of inhomogeneity. For example, acute confluent bronchopneumonia, which typically produces homogeneous segmental consolidation, may cavitate and thus create a shadow of relative inhomogeneity; such disease clearly is different pathogenetically from postprimary tuberculosis, in which cavitation accentuates an already inhomogeneous pattern.

TABLE 3
Inhomogeneous Opacities Without Recognizable Segmental Distribution

Etiology	Loss of Volume	Anatomic Distribution	Additional Findings	Comments
DEVELOPMENTAL Congenital cystic adenomatoid malformation	None	———	Tends to expand involved hemithorax. Mass contains numerous irregular air-containing cysts.	Seen predominantly in infants; mass communicates with bronchial tree and is supplied by the pulmonary circulation. (*See* page 719.)
INFECTIOUS **Bacteria** *Mycobacterium tuberculosis.*	0	Apical and posterior portion of upper lobes (rarely anterior alone); superior portion of lower lobes.	Cavitation not infrequent; effusion and lymph node enlargement rare.	Postprimary tuberculosis. (*See* pages 911 and 938.)
Pseudomonas pseudomallei.	+ to + + +	Predominantly upper lobes.	Frequently associated with cavitation.	Resembles postprimary tuberculosis. Has been described as "unresolved pneumonia" and is the chronic form of the disease. (*See* page 860.)
Klebsiella-Enterobacter-Serratia species.	+ to + + +	Predominantly upper lobes.	May be associated with cavitation.	The chronic phase of the disease; closely simulates pulmonary tuberculosis. (*See* page 846.)
Bacillus anthracis.	0	No known predilection.	Mediastinal lymph node enlargement predominant finding.	Opacities due to pulmonary hemorrhage, not to pneumonia. (*See* page 842.)

Fungi

Paracoccidioides (*Blastomyces*) *brasiliensis.*	0	Lower lobe predominance.	Hilar node enlargement variable.	Progressive disease indistinguishable in pattern from postprimary tuberculosis except for lobar predominance. (*See* page 975.)
Histoplasma capsulatum.	0	Primary infection commonly in lower lobes; postprimary disease usually in upper lobes.	In primary disease, hilar lymph node enlargement frequent; pleural effusion may be present but is not common. In postprimary disease, cavitation may be present, but as with postprimary tuberculosis, hilar lymph node enlargement is uncommon. In postprimary disease, a calcified focus elsewhere in the lungs is frequently present, similar to Ranke's complex of primary tuberculosis.	There are no clear-cut distinguishing roentgenographic features from primary or postprimary tuberculosis. (*See* page 853.)
Coccidioides immitis.	0	Upper lobes.	Densities may be "fleeting" in character and may leave behind thin-walled cavities.	This is the so-called benign form of the disease and generally does not produce symptoms. (*See* page 962.)
Blastomyces dermatitidis.	0	Upper lobe predominance in ratio of 3:2.	Cavitation in 15 per cent of cases; bone involvement in 25 per cent, either by direct extension across pleura or by bloodstream. Pleural effusion and lymph node enlargement rare.	(*See* page 970.)

Viruses and Mycoplasma

All viruses listed in Table 4.	0	Predominantly lower lobes.	None.	A specific segmental distribution may not be recognizable at certain stages of these acute pneumonias.

23

Table continued on following page

TABLE 3
Inhomogeneous Opacities Without Recognizable Segmental Distribution *(Continued)*

Etiology	Loss of Volume	Anatomic Distribution	Additional Findings	Comments
IMMUNOLOGIC Löffler's syndrome.	0	Peripheral lung zones without upper or lower predilection.	Consolidation generally ill-defined and transitory or migratory in character.	Consolidation more characteristically homogeneous. Eosinophilia invariable. (*See* page 1291.)
TRAUMATIC Chronic irradiation fibrosis; irradiation pneumonitis.	+ + + to + + + +	Generally corresponds to the area irradiated.	Characteristically there is obliteration of all architectural markings owing to replacement with fibrous tissue. Dense fibrotic strands frequently extend from the hilum to the periphery.	Differentiation from lymphangitic spread of carcinoma may be difficult if changes are bilateral although lack of progression over a period of time should permit differentiation. Acute irradiation pneumonitis characteristically produces a homogeneous nonsegmental pattern (*see* Table 1) but in some cases it is inhomogeneous. (*See* page 2551.)
IDIOPATHIC Ankylosing spondylitis and upper lobe pulmonary fibrosis.	+ + + to + + + +	Uniquely upper lobes.	Bone and joint manifestations of ankylosing spondylitis.	Cavitation is fairly frequent and may be associated with mycetoma formation. (*See* page 1208.)

24

TABLE 4

Inhomogeneous Opacities of Recognizable Segmental Distribution

This pattern characterizes bronchopneumonia or "lobular" pneumonia. The infection is propagated distally in the bronchovascular bundles and thus invariably is of segmental distribution. The parenchymal changes consist of a combination of focal consolidation, atelectasis, and overinflation, resulting in an inhomogeneous roentgenographic pattern. Bronchiectasis produces the same appearance.

TABLE 4
Inhomogeneous Opacities of Recognizable Segmental Distribution

Etiology	Loss of Volume	Anatomic Distribution	Additional Findings	Comments
INFECTIOUS				
Bacteria				
Haemophilus influenzae.	+ to + +	Predominantly lower lobes.	Pleural effusion common.	Typical roentgenographic pattern of bronchopneumonia. (*See* page 853.)
Streptococcus pneumoniae.	+ to + +	Dependent portions of upper or lower lobes.	Often in disabled hospitalized patients with COPD.	Atypical presentation. Conforms to the usual pattern of acute bronchopneumonia. (*See* page 833.)
Mycobacterium tuberculosis (postprimary).	+ to + + +	Apical and posterior segments upper lobes; superior segment lower lobes.	Frequently associated with tuberculous bronchiectasis and sometimes with cavitation.	Chronic stage of the disease, usually fibrotic (but not necessarily inactive). (*See* pages 911 and 938.)
Salmonella species. *Brucella* species. *Staphylococcus aureus.* *Streptococcus pyogenes.* *Haemophilus pertussis.* *Klebsiella-Enterobacter-Serratia* genera.	+ to + +	Predominantly lower lobes.	Variable with specific organism.	On rare occasions, any of these organisms may give rise to an inhomogeneous segmental pattern.

26

Fungi

Histoplasma capsulatum.	+ to + + +	Upper lobes.	——	Indistinguishable in appearance from chronic postprimary tuberculosis. (*See* page 953.)
Candida albicans.	+ to + +	No predilection.	May be associated with cavitation.	This pattern of bronchopneumonia is the usual method of presentation. (*See* page 987.)
Mucorales order (including *Mucor* species). *Sporothrix schenckii.*	+ to + +	No known predilection.	——	Bronchopneumonia. (*See* pages 1016 and 1019.)

Viruses

Mycoplasma pneumoniae.	0	Predominantly lower lobes.	Pleural effusion and lymph node enlargement rare in adults. Hilar lymph node enlargement found in 25 per cent of children.	Characteristic reticular pattern with superimposed patchy areas of airspace consolidation. Generally indistinguishable from viral pneumonitis. (*See* page 1038.)
Influenza. Adenoviruses. Psittacosis (ornithosis). Parainfluenza. Coxsackie.	0	Predominantly lower lobes.	Hilar lymph node enlargement is seen in some patients with ornithosis.	Roentgenographic pattern indistinguishable within the group and indistinguishable from that of *Mycoplasma* pneumonia.

27

Table continued on following page

TABLE 4
Inhomogeneous Opacities of Recognizable Segmental Distribution *(Continued)*

Etiology	Loss of Volume	Anatomic Distribution	Additional Findings	Comments
INFECTIOUS *(Continued)* **Viruses** *(Continued)* ECHO. Rubeola.	0	Predominantly lower lobes.	Hilar lymph node enlargement frequent.	In measles this pattern is probably due to superimposed bacterial bronchopneumonia. *(See* pages 1050 and 1056.)
Respiratory syncytial.	0	Predominantly lower lobes.	Diffuse overinflation secondary to bronchitis and bronchiolitis.	Characteristically a disease of infants and young children, but may occur in adults. *(See* page 1049.)
Parasites *Toxoplasma gondii.*	0	No predilection.	Hilar lymph node enlargement common.	*(See* page 1081.)
IMMUNOLOGIC Systemic lupus erythematosus.	Progressive loss of lung volume may be characteristic but is unrelated to roentgenographic evidence of localized pulmonary disease.	Commonly peripherally situated in the lung bases.	Cardiac enlargement in 35 to 50 per cent of patients, commonly due to pericardial effusion. Bilateral pleural effusion common.	Pulmonary change is nonspecific, generally in form of basal pneumonitis or focal atelectasis. *(See* page 1189.)

28

NEOPLASTIC

Hodgkin's disease.	0	No predilection.	Mediastinal and hilar lymph node enlargement almost invariable. Kerley lines in some cases. Pleural effusion in 30 per cent of cases.	The most common form of pulmonary parenchymal involvement. Results from direct extension from mediastinal and hilar nodes along interstitial tissues. (*See* page 1507.)
All endobronchial neoplasms, either benign or malignant.	0 to + + + +	No predilection.	——	In any situation where a neoplasm has resulted in obstructive pneumonitis, the partial relief of the obstruction during therapy may permit visualization of air-containing distorted channels within the obstructed segment.

Table continued on following page

Etiology	Loss of Volume	Anatomic Distribution	Additional Findings	Comments
INHALATIONAL				
Chronic aspiration.	+ to + + +	Posterior segments of lower or upper lobes; on serial roentgenographic examinations, anatomic distribution may vary considerably.	Almost always associated with underlying condition such as Zenker's diverticulum, esophageal stenosis, achalasia, or disturbances in swallowing of neuromuscular origin.	The roentgenographic picture suggests typical "bronchopneumonia." Multiple segments may be involved. Bronchiectasis may develop in involved segments. *(See page 2387.)*
Aspiration of solid foreign bodies.	+ to + +	Almost exclusively lower lobes, the ratio of right to left being 2:1.	The foreign body is radiopaque in approximately 10 per cent of cases.	The pattern is purely segmental and is produced by a combination of atelectasis and pneumonitis secondary to bronchial obstruction. May be associated with bronchiectasis. *(See page 2382.)*
Lipoid pneumonia.	0 to +	Dependent portions of upper and lower lobes (occasionally right middle lobe or lingula).	CT can sometimes reveal the fatty nature of the opacity.	A reticular pattern may develop as a result of the movement of oil (in macrophages) from the airspaces into the interstitial tissues. *(See page 2398.)*
AIRWAYS DISEASE				
Bronchiectasis.	+ to + + +	More frequent in lower lobes and right middle lobe. Multiple segments or lobes may be involved.	Saccular bronchiectasis may show fluid levels. Compensatory overinflation may be present in unaffected lung.	*(See page 2186.)*

TABLE 5

Cystic and Cavitary Disease

This table includes all forms of pulmonary disease characterized by circumscribed air-containing spaces with distinct walls. This broad definition includes such entities as blebs, bullae, and cystic bronchiectasis. Air-fluid levels may be present or absent. Cavities may be single or multiple.

Table 5
Cystic and Cavitary Disease

Etiology	Anatomic Distribution	Character of Wall	Additional Findings	Comments
DEVELOPMENTAL				
Intralobar bronchopulmonary sequestration.	Two thirds of cases left lower lobe, one third right lower lobe. Almost invariably contiguous to diaphragm.	May be thin- or thick-walled.	Air-fluid levels may be present. The cyst volume may change on serial roentgenographic examinations. Cyst may be masked by pneumonia in surrounding parenchyma.	Cyst may be solitary but more commonly multilocular or multiple. (*See* page 702.)
Bronchial cyst.	Medial third of lower lobes.	Thin-walled.	An air-fluid level may be present. When pneumonitis leads to communication between cyst and the bronchial tree, the cavity may be masked by the surrounding pneumonia.	75 per cent of bronchial cysts eventually become air-containing as a result of communication with contiguous lung. (*See* page 712.)
Congenital adenomatoid malformation.	No definite predilection.	Multiple air-containing cysts scattered irregularly through a mass of unit density.	An expanding process, causing enlargement of affected lung and hemithorax.	Volume of lung affected varies considerably. (*See* page 719.)
INFECTIOUS				
Bacteria				
Staphylococcus aureus.	No lobar predilection.	Tends to be thick with ragged inner lining.	Pleural effusion (empyema) with or without bronchopleural fistula (pyopneumothorax) almost invariable in children and may occur in adults.	In adults, cavities result from tissue necrosis; in children, air-containing spaces commonly due to pneumatocele formation. Staphylococcal pyemia may lead to multiple small abscesses widely distributed throughout both lungs. (*See* page 836.)

32

Klebsiela-Enterobacter-Serratic species.	Upper lobes predominate.	Tends to be thick with ragged inner lining.	Pleural effusion (empyema) may be present. Cavity rarely contains large masses of necrotic lung — acute lung gangrene.	Abscess formation in acute pneumonia. Cavities are usually single but tend to be multilocular. Multiple cavities may be present if pneumonia is multilobar. (*See* page 846.)
Mycobacterium species.	Apical and posterior regions of upper lobes and apical region of lower lobes.	Tends to be of moderate thickness. Inner lining generally smooth.	Cavities may be multiple.	Cavitation tends to be a more prominent feature of atypical mycobacterial disease than of *Mycobacterium tuberculosis* infection. (*See* pages 913 and 938.)
Pseudomonas aeruginosa. Escherichia coli.	Predominantly lower lobes.	Highly variable.	Empyema frequent.	Often the result of bacteremia from an extrathoracic focus (GU tract). Tends to occur in debilitated states (alcoholism or diabetes). (*See* page 855.)
Streptococcus pneumoniae.	Upper lobe predilection.	Thick, with ragged inner lining.	The cavity may contain large irregular masses of necrotic lung — acute lung gangrene.	A rare complication of fulminating pneumococcal pneumonia. (*See* page 831.)
Pseudomonas pseudomallei.	Upper lobes predominate.	Moderately thick.	Effusions rare.	(*See* page 860.)
Anaerobic organisms.	Posterior portion of both lungs.	Tends to be thick with ragged inner lining.	Cavities frequently multiple. Empyema common.	Tend to be associated with debilitation, alcoholism, and poor oral hygiene. (*See* page 875.)
Actinomyces israelii. Nocardia species.	Lower lobe predilection, bilateral.	Generally thick-walled.	Pleural effusion (empyema) is common as is extension into the chest wall with or without rib destruction.	Roentgenographic patterns in infections with these two organisms are indistinguishable. (*See* pages 1024 and 1028.)

33

Table continued on following page

Table 5
Cystic and Cavitary Disease (Continued)

Etiology	Anatomic Distribution	Character of Wall	Additional Findings	Comments
INFECTIOUS (Continued)				
Fungi				
Histoplasma capsulatum.	Predominantly upper lobes.	Variable.	Cavities may be multiple.	No clear-cut distinguishing roentgenographic features from postprimary tuberculosis. (See page 953.)
Coccidioides immitis.	Predominantly upper lobes.	Tends to be very thin-walled.	These thin-walled cavities tend to occur in the asymptomatic form of the disease following "fleeting" pneumonitis.	Not to be confused with cavitating nodules, which tend to be somewhat thicker-walled and frequently multiple. (See page 962.)
Blastomyces dermatitidis.	No predilection.	Variable, but generally thick-walled.	Cavitation occurs in about 15 per cent of cases. Pleural effusion and hilar lymph node enlargement very uncommon.	(See page 970.)
Cryptococcus neoformans.	Predominantly lower lobes.	Variable, but generally thick-walled.	Cavitation occurs in about 15 per cent of cases. Pleural effusion and hilar lymph node enlargement very uncommon.	(See page 977.)
Geotrichum species. Sporothrix schenckii. }	Upper lobe predilection.	Characteristically thin-walled.	———	(See pages 1018 and 1019.)
Mucorales order.	Not distinctive.	———	———	(See page 1016.)

34

Aspergillus species.	——	——	——	The invasive form of the disease is often associated with cavitation. (*See* page 1007.)
Parasite:				
Entamoeba histolytica (amebiasis).	Almost restricted to right lower lobe.	Generally thick-walled with irregular ragged inner lining.	Right pleural effusion almost invariable.	Organisms enter thorax via right hemidiaphragm from liver abscess. (*See* page 1081.)
Paragonimus westermani.	No predilection.	Characteristically thin-walled, with local elevation or hump on inner lining.	In addition to cavities, there may be isolated nodular shadows containing vacuoles. Pleural effusion rarely.	Organisms enter thorax via diaphragm from peritoneal space. (*See* page 1109.)
Echinococcus granulosus (hydatid cyst).	Lower lobe predilection.	Air may dissect between ectocyst and endocyst, creating a halo; or contents of cyst may be expelled into bronchial tree, leaving a thin-walled cystic space.	Irregularities of fluid layer caused by collapsed membranes (water-lily sign or sign of the camalote). Hydropneumothorax occasionally.	(*See* page 1102.)
Pneumocystis carinii.	Upper lobe predilection.	Thin-walled.	Typical widespread interstitial/airspace disease; pneumothorax frequent.	This pattern is occurring with increasing frequency in patients with AIDS. (*See* page 1085.)
IMMUNOLOGIC				
Wegener's granulomatosis.	Widely distributed and bilateral, with no predilection for upper or lower lung zones.	Usually thick, with irregular inner lining. In time, cavities may become thin-walled cystic spaces.	Cavities commonly multiple but all masses do not necessarily cavitate.	Cavitation occurs eventually in from one third to one half of patients. With treatment, cavitary lesions may disappear or heal with scar formation. (*See* page 1241.)

35

Table continued on following page

Table 5
Cystic and Cavitary Disease *(Continued)*

Etiology	Anatomic Distribution	Character of Wall	Additional Findings	Comments
IMMUNOLOGIC *(Continued)*				
Rheumatoid (necrobiotic) nodule.	Peripheral subpleural parenchyma, commonly in lower lobes.	Thick with smooth inner lining. With remission of the arthritis, cavities may become thin-walled and gradually disappear.	Pleural effusion or spontaneous pneumothorax.	Well-circumscribed masses are more frequently multiple than solitary and range in size from 3 mm to 7 cm. Cavitary nodules wax and wane in concert with frequently associated subcutaneous nodules. (*See* page 1211.)
NEOPLASTIC				
Pulmonary carcinoma.	Clear-cut predilection for upper lobes, both lungs being affected equally.	Tends to be thick, with an irregular, nodular inner lining (mural nodules). Thin-walled cavities simulating bronchial cysts occur occasionally.	Chunks of necrotic cancer occasionally may become detached and lie free within the cavity, simulating fungus ball.	Cavitation occurs in 2 to 10 per cent of pulmonary carcinomas, most commonly in lesions peripherally located. The majority are squamous-cell in type (adenocarcinomas and large cell carcinomas cavitate occasionally, small cell carcinomas rarely if ever). (*See* page 1411.)
Hematogenous metastases.	Cavitation occurs more frequently in upper than in lower lobe lesions.	May be thin- or thick-walled.	Cavitation may involve only a few of multiple nodules throughout the lungs, such nodules characteristically showing considerable variation in size.	Cavitation in metastatic neoplasms less common (4 per cent) than in primary neoplasms (9 per cent). Occurs more frequently in squamous cell neoplasms but also in adenocarcinoma (particularly from the large bowel) and sarcoma. (*See* page 1628.)

Hodgkin's disease.	Lower lobe predilection.	Thin- or thick-walled.	Cavities are frequently multiple. Commonly associated with mediastinal and hilar lymph node enlargement.	Cavitation occurs characteristically in peripheral parenchymal consolidation. (*See* page 1508.)
THROMBOEMBOLIC				
Septic embolism.	Lower lobe predilection, predominantly posterior and lateral segments.	Usually thin-walled but may be thick, with shaggy inner lining.	Prominent feeding artery, associated pleural effusion, raised diaphragm, or multiple lesions may suggest the diagnosis. A mass of necrotic lung may separate and lie within the cavity, simulating fungus ball.	A rare manifestation which may be misdiagnosed unless clinical picture and associated roentgenographic findings suggest the possibility. Cavitation can also occur as a result of bacterial superinfection of a bland infarct. (*See* page 1751.)
INHALATIONAL				
Silicosis – large opacities (progressive massive fibrosis).	Strong predilection for upper lobes.	Tends to be thick with irregular inner lining.	Background of nodular or reticulonodular disease is inevitable although serial examinations may reveal diminution in the number of nodules due to incorporation into the massive consolidation. Hilar lymph node enlargement is the rule, with or without eggshell calcification.	Cavitation in conglomerate lesions can be the result of either superimposed tuberculosis or ischemic necrosis. (*See* page 2289.)
Coal workers' pneumoconiosis – large opacities (progressive massive fibrosis).	Strong predilection for upper lobes.	Tends to be thick with irregular inner lining.	Background of simple coal workers' pneumoconiosis throughout the remainder of the lungs.	Cavitation in conglomerate shadows can be caused by either superimposed tuberculosis or ischemic necrosis. (*See* page 2313.)

Table continued on following page

Table 5
Cystic and Cavitary Disease *(Continued)*

Etiology	Anatomic Distribution	Character of Wall	Additional Findings	Comments
AIRWAYS DISEASE				
Blebs or bullae.	Predilection for upper lobes, particularly extreme apex.	Thin-walled.	With infection, fluid levels may develop. In some cases, roentgenologic evidence of diffuse emphysema will be present.	The thinness of the wall is the main differentiating feature from true cavitation. *(See page 2166.)*
Cystic bronchiectasis.	Predilection for lower lobes.	Thin-walled.	Usually considerable loss of volume of affected segment or segments.	"Cavities" represent severely dilated segmental bronchi. Usually multiple and commonly with air-fluid levels. *(See page 2186.)*
TRAUMATIC				
Pulmonary parenchymal laceration (traumatic lung cyst).	Characteristically in the peripheral subpleural parenchyma immediately underlying the point of maximum injury.	Typically thin-walled.	The presence of laceration may be masked by surrounding pulmonary contusion. In some cases of bullet wounds of the lung, a central radiolucency may be observed along the course of the bullet track, simulating a cavity when viewed in the same direction as the wound.	Approximately half these lesions present as thin-walled air-filled cavities (with or without air-fluid levels) and the remainder as pulmonary hematomas. They may be single or multiple, unilocular or multilocular; they are oval or spherical in shape and range from 2 to 14 cm in diameter. *(See page 2481.)*
IDIOPATHIC				
Sarcoidosis.	No predilection.	No typical characteristics.	Cavities may contain mycetomas.	True cavitation in sarcoidosis is rare. Important to exclude all other causes of cavitation before accepting the diagnosis. *(See page 2611.)*

TABLE 6

Solitary Pulmonary Nodules
Less Than 3 cm in Diameter

For the purposes of this table, the criteria for inclusion in this category are as follows:

1. The presence of a solitary roentgenographic shadow not exceeding 3 cm in its largest diameter.

2. The lesion is fairly discrete but not necessarily sharply defined.

3. It may have any contour (smooth, lobulated, or umbilicated) or shape.

4. It may be calcified or cavitated.

5. Satellite lesions may be present.

6. The lesion is surrounded by air-containing lung; *or* if it is adjacent to the visceral pleural surface over the convexity of the thorax, at least two thirds of its circumference is contiguous to air-containing lung.

7. Symptoms may be present.

TABLE 6
Solitary Pulmonary Nodules Less Than 3 cm in Diameter

Etiology	Incidence	Location	Shape	Calcification	Cavitation	Comments
DEVELOPMENTAL Pulmonary bronchial cyst.	Peak incidence third decade; predilection for males and Yemenite Jews.	Lower lobe predilection, most commonly medial third.	Round or oval, smooth, well defined.	Rarely in wall; calcium has been reported in cyst contents.	Yes, when communication occurs with bronchial tree.	Cysts are homogeneous until communication established with contiguous lung, usually because of infection (occurs eventually in 75 per cent of cases). (*See* page 712.)
Pulmonary arteriovenous fistula.	0.6 per cent of Bateson's series. In two thirds of cases, lesions are single.	More common in lower lobes.	Round or oval, slightly lobulated, sharply defined.	Occasionally, probably due to phleboliths.	No.	Diagnosis by identification of feeding artery and draining vein. Angiography of *both lungs* imperative if surgery is contemplated in order to identify multiple fistulae not visible on plain roentgenograms. 40 to 65 per cent of cases have hereditary hemorrhagic telangiectasia. (*See* page 752.)

Varicosity of a pulmonary vein.	Very rare (47 cases reported by 1976).	Medial third of lung (lingular vein on left or medial basal pulmonary vein on right).	Round or oval, lobulated, well defined.	No.	No.	Change in size with Valsalva and Mueller procedures. Differential diagnosis from arteriovenous fistula by late filling and slow drainage on pulmonary angiography. (*See* page 742.)
Congenital bronchial atresia with mucoid impaction.	Very rare.	Strong predilection for the apicoposterior bronchus of the left upper lobe.	Oval, smooth, sharply defined.	No.	No.	The mass consists of inspissated mucus which accumulates within the bronchus immediately distal to the point of obliteration; the lung parenchyma distal to the occlusion is overinflated owing to collateral air drift. (*See* page 721.)

Table continued on following page

Etiology	Incidence	Location	Shape	Calcification	Cavitation	Comments
INFECTIOUS						
Bacteria						
Mycobacterium tuberculosis (tuberculoma).	Common.	Predilection for upper lobes, the right more often than the left.	Round or oval; 25 per cent are lobulated.	Frequent.	Uncommon.	"Satellite" lesions in 80 per cent; the draining bronchus may show irregular thickening of its wall or occasionally bronchostenosis. (*See* pages 923 and 938.)
Fungi						
Histoplasma capsulatum (histoplasmoma).	Common.	More frequently in the lower than in the upper lobes.	Round or oval; typically sharply circumscribed.	Common, often central in location, thus producing the "target" appearance.	Rare.	"Satellite" lesions fairly common. Histoplasmomas may be multiple, varying considerably in size. Associated hilar lymph node calcification is common. (*See* page 949.)
Coccidioides immitis.	Rare.	Upper lobe predilection.	Round or oval; typically sharply circumscribed.	In some cases.	Common; may be thin- or thick-walled.	(*See* page 962.)

Aspergillus species (mucoid impaction).	Very uncommon; largely restricted to patients with bronchospasm.	Upper lobe predilection.	Tends to be finger-like but may be Y-shaped or V-shaped in conformity with bronchial subdivision.	No.	Air-fluid levels may be visible within the markedly dilated bronchus, simulating cavitation.	The mass is caused by mucoid impaction within a proximal segmental bronchus. It tends to be transient in nature, although it may persist unchanged for weeks or even months, or may increase in size while under observation. When the lesion clears, it leaves as a residuum cylindrical or saccular dilatation of the affected bronchi. The impacted bronchus may or may not cause atelectasis of the involved segment; atelectasis frequently is prevented by collateral air drift. (*See* page 993.)
Aspergillus species (mycetoma)	Uncommon.	Upper lobe predilection.	Round or oval.	No.	Invariably situated *within* a cavity.	This is only one of several fungi capable of forming an intracavitary "fungus ball." (*See* page 991.)

Table continued on following page

Etiology	Incidence	Location	Shape	Calcification	Cavitation	Comments
INFECTIOUS *(Continued)* **Parasites** *Echinococcus* (hydatid cyst).	Common in endemic areas.	Lower lobe predilection, right more often than left.	Almost always well circumscribed. Tendency to bizarre, irregular shape.	Very rare.	Common.	*(See* page 1102.)
Dirofilaria immitis.	Rare.	No known predilection.	Well defined.	No.	Sometimes.	Involvement of larger pulmonary arteries may result in a shadow simulating pulmonary infarction. *(See* page 1100.)
IMMUNOLOGIC Rheumatoid (necrobiotic) nodule.	Rare.	In the peripheral subpleural zone, usually lower lobes.	Well defined, smooth.	No.	Common. Cavities possess thick walls and smooth inner lining.	More commonly multiple than solitary. Pleural effusion may be present. Eosinophilia in some patients. Nodules wax and wane in concert with the frequently associated subcutaneous nodules and in proportion to the activity of the rheumatoid arthritis. *(See* page 1211.)

44

Wegener's granulomatosis.	Rare.	No predilection.	Tend to be well defined.	No.	In one third to one half of cases.	Much less common manifestation than multiple nodules, although solitary nodules were observed in 4 of 20 cases in one series. (*See* page 1241.)

NEOPLASTIC

Pulmonary carcinoma.	Varies widely; in patients referred for resection, approximately 40 per cent of solitary nodules will be malignant.	Predominantly upper lobes.	Margins tend to be ill-defined, lobulated, or umbilicated.	Very rare.	2 to 10 per cent.	Satellite lesions very uncommon. (*See* pages 1383 and 1461.)
Carcinoid tumor.	Incidence compared to pulmonary carcinoma 1:50. 20 to 25 per cent of all carcinoid tumors present as solitary nodules.	Predilection for right upper and middle lobes and lingula.	Round or oval, sharply defined, slightly lobulated.	Rare.	Rare.	The remaining 75 to 80 per cent of carcinoid tumors relate to a bronchial lumen and lead to segmental atelectasis or obstructive pneumonitis. (*See* page 1477.)

Table continued on following page

Etiology	Incidence	Location	Shape	Calcification	Cavitation	Comments
NEOPLASTIC *(Continued)* Hamartoma.	Constitute approximately 5 per cent of solitary peripheral nodules.	No lobar predilection.	Well defined; more often lobulated than smooth in a ratio of 2:1.	Incidence varies widely in reported series, but certainly occurs in a minority of cases. "Popcorn" configuration virtually diagnostic.	No.	10 per cent arise endobronchially and then may cause bronchial obstruction, atelectasis, or obstructive pneumonitis. Serial examination may reveal slow growth. (*See* page 1608.)
Neoplasms of muscle, vascular tissue, bone and cartilage, neural tissue, adipose tissues, fibrohistiocytic tissue, and mixed mesenchymal tissue. Miscellaneous neoplasms of uncertain histogenesis. Miscellaneous tumors of non-neoplastic or uncertain nature.	Very rare.	No definite predilection.	Usually well defined.	Rarely.	No.	Rarely these neoplasms may arise within a bronchial wall and thus be manifested roentgenographically by bronchial obstruction and peripheral atelectasis or obstructive pneumonitis. (*See* pages 1577 to 1608.)

46

Hematogenous metastasis.	3 to 5 per cent of asymptomatic nodules.	Predominantly lower lobes.	Smooth or slightly lobulated. Tend to be well defined.	Rarely and only in osteogenic sarcoma or chondrosarcoma.	Occasionally.	In 25 per cent of cases, metastatic lesions to the lungs are solitary. (*See* page 1628.)
Bronchiolo-alveolar carcinoma.	The most common method of presentation of this neoplasm.	No predilection.	Round, smooth, or lobulated; may be sharply or ill-defined.	No.	Rarely.	An air bronchogram or air bronchiologram is a common roentgenographic feature, except in the smaller lesions. Tends to be very slow growing. (*See* page 1414.)
Non-Hodgkin's lymphoma.	Rare.	No predilection.	Round, ovoid, triangular or polyhedral; tends to have fuzzy outline.	No.	In large cell lymphoma, "cyst-like" lesions may occur that resemble cavitation.	May be a manifestation of either primary or secondary disease. (*See* page 1535.)
Multiple myeloma (plasmacytoma).	Rare.	No predilection.	Lobulated.	No.	No.	No distinguishing features from those of peripheral pulmonary carcinoma. (*See* page 1558.)

Table continued on following page

Etiology	Incidence	Location	Shape	Calcification	Cavitation	Comments
TRAUMATIC Pulmonary hematoma.	Uncommon.	Usually in a peripheral subpleural location.	Oval or round, sharply defined, smooth.	No.	A hematoma occurs as a result of hemorrhage into a pulmonary parenchymal laceration or traumatic lung cyst — thus, an air-fluid level may be present as a result of communication with the bronchial tree.	Generally undergo slow but progressive decrease in size, although they may persist for long periods of time, sometimes up to 4 months. May be multiple. Not uncommonly result from segmental or wedge resection of lung parenchyma. The presence of a hematoma may be masked by surrounding pulmonary contusion. *(See* page 2481.)
METABOLIC Bronchopulmonary amyloidosis.	Extremely rare.	No predilection.	——	Occasionally in the periphery.	Occasionally.	*(See* page 2578.)

TABLE 7

Solitary Pulmonary Masses 3 cm or More in Diameter

The general characteristics of lesions included in this table are the same as for solitary nodules less than 3 cm in diameter.

The separation of a group of entities into this category on the basis of size alone is perhaps arbitrary but appears to be necessary in view of the restriction on size imposed by most authorities for inclusion of solitary nodules as so-called coin lesions.

TABLE 7
Solitary Pulmonary Masses 3 cm or More in Diameter

Etiology	Location	Shape	Calcification	Cavitation	Comments
DEVELOPMENTAL					
Intralobar bronchopulmonary sequestration.	Two thirds of cases left lower lobe; one third of cases right lower lobe; rare elsewhere. Almost invariably contiguous to diaphragm in posterior bronchopulmonary segment.	Round, oval, or triangular in shape and typically well defined.	No.	Frequent.	Enclosed within visceral pleura of affected lung. Although cystic in nature, mass remains homogeneous until communication established with contiguous lung as a result of infection. Supplied by systemic artery and drains via pulmonary veins. (*See* page 702.)
Extralobar bronchopulmonary sequestration.	Related to left hemidiaphragm in 90 per cent of cases, lying immediately above, below, or within it.	Well-defined homogeneous mass.	No.	Seldom.	Frequently associated with other anomalies and sometimes with diaphragmatic eventration. Enclosed within its own visceral pleural layer — therefore seldom infected or air-containing (*cf.* intralobar). Supplied by systemic artery (usually from abdominal aorta) and drains via systemic rather than pulmonary veins (IVC or azygos system). (*See* page 709.)

Pulmonary bronchial cyst.	Lower lobe predilection, usually in medial third.	Round or oval.	Rarely in wall.	Only after they have become infected.	Incidence of mediastinal and pulmonary cysts varies, the former predominating in some series and the latter in others. Infection occurs eventually in 75 per cent of cases. (*See* page 712.)
Congenital adenomatoid malformation.	No lobar predominance.	Round or oval.	No.	See comments.	The solid form is much less common than the cystic. Manifested as a large, space-occupying homogeneous mass. (*See* page 719.)

INFECTIOUS

Acute or chronic lung abscess.	Predilection for posterior portions of upper or lower lobes.	Tends to be round; somewhat ill-defined when acute but sharply defined when chronic.	No.	Almost inevitable.	Usually of staphylococcal or anaerobic etiology. The mass may remain unchanged for many weeks without perforation into bronchial tree. (*See* pages 836 and 875.)
Cryptococcus neoformans.	Lower lobe predominance, usually in the periphery.	Tends to be well defined, homogeneous in density, and solitary.	No.	Reported in 16 per cent of cases.	Commonly pleural based. (*See* page 977.)

51

Table continued on following page

TABLE 7
Solitary Pulmonary Masses 3 cm or More in Diameter *(Continued)*

Etiology	Location	Shape	Calcification	Cavitation	Comments
INFECTIOUS *(Continued)* *Blastomyces dermatitidis.*	No lobar predominance.	Margins tend to be ill-defined.	No.	Uncommon.	Frequency of this manifestation varies widely in reported series. May simulate pulmonary carcinoma. *(See* page 970.)
Nocardia asteroides.	Lower lobe predominance.	Indistinguishable from actinomycosis.	No.	Frequent.	The initial roentgenographic presentation in 4 of 12 cases in one series, with cavitation in all. *(See* page 1028.)
Actinomyces israelii.	Lower lobe predominance.	Somewhat ill-defined. Simulates pulmonary carcinoma.	No.	Frequent.	The initial roentgenographic presentation in 6 of 15 cases in one series. *(See* page 1024.)
Coccidioides immitis.	Lower lobe predominance.	Round or oval.	No.	Uncommon.	Can simulate a peripheral pulmonary carcinoma. *(See* page 958.)
Echinococcus granulosus (hydatid cyst).	Predilection for lower lobes, right more often than left.	Sharply defined; tends to possess bizarre, irregular shape.	Extremely rare.	Common.	Communication with bronchial tree may produce the "meniscus" sign or sign of the camalote. *(See* page 1102.)

52

IMMUNOLOGIC

Wegener's granulomatosis.	No predilection.	Well circumscribed.	No.	In one third to one half of cases.	Solitary nodules much less common than multiple. Range from a few millimeters to 9 cm in diameter. The lesion was solitary in 4 of 20 cases in one series. (*See* page 1241.)

NEOPLASTIC

Pulmonary carcinoma.	Predominantly upper lobes.	Margins tend to be ill-defined, lobulated, or umbilicated.	No.	Fairly common.	Most common method of presentation of large cell carcinoma, somewhat less common in adenocarcinoma and squamous-cell carcinoma and very uncommon in small cell carcinoma. (*See* pages 1342 and 1367.)
All neoplasms of soft tissue bone, and cartilage listed in Table 6.	No definite predilection.	Well defined, smooth.	Rarely.	No.	Any of these neoplasms may reach a large size.
Hematogenous metastasis.	Predominantly lower lobes.	Tend to be sharply defined, somewhat lobulated.	Rare — restricted to metastatic osteogenic sarcoma or chondrosarcoma.	Predominantly in upper lobe lesions but is uncommon.	(*See* page 1625.)

53

Table continued on following page

TABLE 7
Solitary Pulmonary Masses 3 cm or More in Diameter *(Continued)*

Etiology	Location	Shape	Calcification	Cavitation	Comments
NEOPLASTIC *(Continued)* Bronchiolo-alveolar carcinoma.	No predilection.	Tends to be ill-defined.	No.	No.	Tends to be very slow growing; may occupy most of the volume of a lobe, but there is no tendency to cross interlobar fissures. Air bronchogram frequent. *(See* page 1414.)
Hodgkin's disease.	No predilection.	Shaggy and ill-defined.	No.	Sometimes.	Size ranges widely and may vary with time. An air bronchogram should be visible. *(See* page 1507.)
Non-Hodgkin's lymphoma.	No clear-cut lobar predilection; tends to be more centrally than peripherally located.	Smooth and fairly sharply defined.	No.	Rare.	May be a manifestation of either primary or secondary lymphoma. The primary form is often without associated hilar or mediastinal lymph node enlargement, and tends to grow slowly. Rarely obstructs the bronchial tree so that an air bronchogram is almost invariable. *(See* page 1535.)

Multiple myeloma (plasmacytoma).	Over the convexity of thorax contiguous to chest wall.	Sharply defined, possessing an obtuse angle with the chest wall.	No.	No.	Due to protrusion into the thorax of a primary lesion originating in a rib—thus almost invariably associated with a destructive lesion of one or more ribs. May reach a very large size. (*See* page 1558.)
INHALATIONAL Lipoid pneumonia.	Dependent portions of upper and lower lobes (occasionally right middle lobe or lingula).	Well defined, smooth or lobulated. Sometimes with very shaggy outer margin.	No.	No.	Usually homogeneous in density. Closely simulates peripheral pulmonary carcinoma. (*See* page 2402.)

Table continued on following page

TABLE 7
Solitary Pulmonary Masses 3 cm or More in Diameter *(Continued)*

Etiology	Location	Shape	Calcification	Cavitation	Comments
INHALATIONAL *(Continued)* Silicosis (progressive massive fibrosis).	Characteristically conglomerate shadows develop in the periphery of the mid or upper lung zones and in time tend to migrate toward the hilum.	Tend to be broader in the sagittal plane than in the coronal. Their margins may be irregular and somewhat ill-defined so as to simulate peripheral pulmonary carcinoma.	No.	Sometimes.	The background pattern of diffuse silicosis may be quite apparent, but the more extensive the progressive massive fibrosis, the less the nodularity apparent in the remainder of the lungs (due to incorporation of nodular lesions into the massive consolidation). Because of cicatrization atelectasis, compensatory overinflation or overt emphysema of remainder of lung is common. Cavitation may occur in conglomerate lesions. Hilar lymph node enlargement is usual and in an occasional case may be associated with "eggshell calcification." *(See* page 2282.)

Coal workers' pneumoconiosis (progressive massive fibrosis).	Marked predilection for upper lobes; tends to originate in the periphery of the lung, migrating toward the hilum over a period of years.	Similar to large opacities of silicosis.	No.	Sometimes.	The background of diffuse nodular or reticulonodular shadows is usually evident, although incorporation of the individual foci into the conglomerate consolidation may render the nodular pattern inconspicuous. Compensatory overinflation or emphysema develops in lower lobes in response to cicatrization atelectasis. (*See* page 2282.)
Asbestosis (large opacities).	Lower zonal predominance in contrast to similar lesions of silicosis and coal workers' pneumoconiosis.	Tend to be smaller than large opacities of silicosis. Round or oval; ill-defined.	No.	No.	Background pattern of diffuse pulmonary asbestosis, usually with pleural thickening, plaques, and calcification. (*See* pages 2316 and 2345.)
Talcosis (large opacities).	Lower zonal predominance.	Variable.	No.	No.	Background pattern of general haziness, nodulation, and reticulation. Pleural plaque formation common. (*See* page 2354.)

57

Table continued on following page

TABLE 7
Solitary Pulmonary Masses 3 cm or More in Diameter *(Continued)*

Etiology	Location	Shape	Calcification	Cavitation	Comments
TRAUMATIC					
Pulmonary hematoma.	Usually deep to point of maximum trauma.	Sharply defined, round or oval.	No.	No.	Hematomas are usually less than 6 cm in diameter but occasionally are very large. Resolution may take several months. (*See* page 2481.)
INCIDENTAL					
Round atelectasis.	Lower zonal predominance.	Round or oval.	No.	No.	Invariably associated with pleural fibrosis and often with asbestos-related pleural disease. (*See* pages 489 and 2328.)

TABLE 8

Multiple Pulmonary Nodules, With or Without Cavitation

The individual lesions generally possess the same characteristics as those described in Tables 6 and 7.

Cavitation or calcification may be present or absent in some or all of the lesions.

TABLE 8
Multiple Pulmonary Nodules, With or Without Cavitation

Etiology	Location	Size and Shape	Calcification	Cavitation	General Comments
DEVELOPMENTAL Pulmonary arteriovenous fistula.	Lower lobe predilection.	One to several centimeters; round or oval, lobulated, well defined.	No.	No.	Multiple in one third of all cases. Diagnosis by identification of feeding artery and draining vein; lesions may change in size between Valsalva and Mueller procedures; angiography necessary to identify all fistulae. 40 to 65 per cent of cases associated with hereditary hemorrhagic telangiectasia. (*See* page 752.)
Varicosities of the pulmonary veins.	Medially, close to left atrium.	1 to 3 cm; round or oval.	No.	No.	May be congenital or acquired. Consists of tortuosity and dilatation of pulmonary veins just before their entrance into the left atrium. Diagnosis by angiography or CT. (*See* page 742.)
INFECTIOUS Pyemic abscesses.	Generalized but more numerous in lower lobes.	Range from 0.5 to 4 cm; usually round and well defined.	No.	Common, usually thick-walled.	Commonly caused by *Staphylococcus aureus*. (*See* page 838.)
Pseudomonas pseudomallei.	No predilection.	4 to 11 mm; irregular and poorly defined.	No.	Common.	Nodules tend to enlarge, coalesce, and cavitate as the disease progresses. (*See* page 860.)

Coccidioides immitis.	Upper lobe predilection.	0.5 to 3.0 cm; round or oval, well defined.	Sometimes.	Common; may be thin- or thick-walled.	In approximately 2 per cent of affected patients, multiple cavities may be associated with pneumothorax and empyema. In contrast to tuberculosis, cavitary disease may occur in anterior segment of an upper lobe. (*See* page 962.)
Histoplasma capsulatum.	No predilection.	0.5 to 3.0 cm; round and sharply defined.	Sometimes.	No.	May remain unchanged over many years or may undergo slow growth. Seldom exceed 4 or 5 in number. (*See* page 949.)
Paragonimus westermani.	Lower lobe predilection, usually in the periphery.	3 to 4 cm; well defined.	Occasionally.	Common.	Multiple ring opacities or thin-walled cysts are characteristic. (*See* page 1109.)

IMMUNOLOGIC

Wegener's granulomatosis.	Widely distributed, bilateral, no predilection for upper or lower lung zones.	5 mm to 9 cm; round, sharply defined.	No.	In one third to one half of patients; characteristically thick-walled, with irregular, shaggy inner lining.	May be associated with focal areas of pneumonitis. Typically occur in patients who manifest no allergic background. Note related but somewhat different condition "allergic granulomatosis." (*See* page 1241.)

Table continued on following page

TABLE 8
Multiple Pulmonary Nodules, With or Without Cavitation *(Continued)*

Etiology	Location	Size and Shape	Calcification	Cavitation	General Comments
IMMUNOLOGIC *(Continued)* Rheumatoid (necrobiotic) nodules.	Peripheral subpleural parenchyma, more commonly lower lobes.	3 mm to 7 cm; round, well defined, smooth.	No.	Common, usually with thick walls and smooth inner lining.	Nodules tend to wax and wane in concert with subcutaneous nodules and in proportion to the activity of the rheumatoid arthritis. With remission of arthritis, cavities may become thin-walled and gradually disappear. In Caplan's syndrome, nodules tend to develop rapidly and appear in crops; both cavitation and calcification may occur in this variety of rheumatoid nodule. *(See* page 1211.)
NEOPLASTIC Tracheobronchial papillomas.	No predilection.	Up to several centimeters; round, sharply defined.	No.	Frequent.	Obstruction of airways leads to peripheral atelectasis and obstructive pneumonitis. Diagnosis is suggested by a combination of multiple solid or cavitary lesions throughout the lungs associated with laryngeal or tracheal papillomas. *(See* page 1502.)
Hematogenous metastases.	Predilection for lower lobes.	3 mm to 6 cm or more; typically round and sharply defined.	Rare, but if present, virtually diagnostic of osteogenic sarcoma or chondrosarcoma.	In approximately 4 per cent of cases, more frequently in upper lobes.	Wide range in size of multiple nodules is highly suggestive of the diagnosis. Seldom associated with mediastinal or bronchopulmonary lymph node enlargement. *(See* page 1625.)

Non-Hodgkin's lymphoma.	More numerous in lower lung zones.	3 mm to 7 cm; round, ovoid, triangular, or polyhedral, usually with fuzzy outlines.	No.	"Cyst-like" lesions may occur in large cell lymphoma, simulating cavitation.	Most often a manifestation of *secondary* lymphoma. Mediastinal and bronchopulmonary lymph node enlargement is associated in some cases. (*See* page 1535.)
Multiple myeloma (plasmacytoma).	No predilection.	Lobulated.	No.	No.	(*See* page 1558.)
THROMBOEMBOLIC Septic emboli.	Lower lobe predilection.	Highly variable; commonly 2 to 6 cm. Round or wedge-shaped.	No.	Frequent, usually with thin walls.	Nodules tend to be peripherally located and ill-defined. May develop a central loose body (the "target sign") representing detached fragments of necrotic lung within a cavity. (*See* page 1751.)
TRAUMATIC Multiple pulmonary hematomas.	Unilateral or bilateral, generally in lung deep to maximum trauma.	Highly variable. Commonly 2 to 6 cm but may be very large. Sharply defined.	No.	No.	Generally undergo slow but progressive decrease in size and may persist for weeks or even months. Initially, hematomas may be masked by surrounding pulmonary contusion. (*See* page 2481.)

Table continued on following page

Etiology	Location	Size and Shape	Calcification	Cavitation	General Comments
METABOLIC Bronchopulmonary amyloidosis.	Widely distributed.	Highly variable.	Lesions may be calcified or ossified.	Sometimes.	This is the parenchymal form of the disease. (*See* page 2578.)
IDIOPATHIC Sarcoidosis.	Widely distributed.	Average diameter greater than 1 cm.	No.	No.	A rare pattern in sarcoidosis (in only 3 of 150 patients in one series). Simulates metastases. (*See* page 2611.)

TABLE 9

**Diffuse Pulmonary Disease
With a Predominantly Acinar Pattern**

"Diffuse" implies involvement of all lobes of both lungs. Although the disease necessarily is widespread, it need not affect all lung regions uniformly. For example, the lower lung zones may be involved to a greater or lesser degree than the upper, or the central and mid portions of the lungs may be more severely affected than the peripheral ("bat's wing" distribution).

The term "acinar pattern" implies airspace consolidation, which may be confluent and thereby render individual acinar shadows unidentifiable.

Other abnormalities such as pleural effusion and cardiac enlargement may be present.

TABLE 9
Diffuse Pulmonary Disease With a Predominantly Acinar Pattern

Etiology	Anatomic Distribution	Volume of Thorax	Additional Findings	Comments
INFECTIOUS				
Histoplasma capsulatum.	Generalized.	Unaffected.	Hilar lymph node enlargement frequent.	Acute widely disseminated histoplasmosis; symptoms may be disproportionately mild. Over a period of years, healing may result in multiple small calcific foci. (*See* page 947.)
Varicella-zoster virus (chickenpox pneumonia).	Widespread; acinar lesions may be confluent in central areas of lungs.	Unaffected.	Hilar lymph node enlargement in some cases.	Over a period of many years, healing may result in multiple small calcific foci throughout the lungs. (*See* page 1062.)
Influenza virus.	Uniform.	Unaffected.	"Mitral configuration" of the heart may be present.	This pattern in acute influenza virus pneumonia occurs particularly in patients who have mitral stenosis or who are pregnant. (*See* page 1043.)
Ascaris lumbricoides or *Ascaris suum.*	Generalized.	Unaffected.	None.	Represents severe edema occasioned by allergic response to the passage of larvae through the pulmonary circulation. (*See* page 1093.)
IMMUNOLOGIC				
Goodpasture's syndrome and idiopathic pulmonary hemorrhage.	Widespread but more prominent in perihilar areas and in mid-lung and lower lung zones.	Unchanged.	Confluence of opacities may occur, in which circumstances an air bronchogram will be seen. Lymph node enlargement may be recognized occasionally.	An acinar pattern is seen in relatively pure form in the early stages of these diseases, but with the accumulation of hemosiderin in interstitial space, the pattern becomes reticular. (*See* page 1181.)

66

Leukocytoclastic vasculitis	Generalized	Unaffected.	None.	Histologic term indicating small vessel vasculitis associated with more or less diffuse airspace hemorrhage. Occurs most frequently with Wegener's granulomatosis and SLE. (*See* page 1264.)
NEOPLASTIC				
Bronchiolo-alveolar carcinoma.	Diffuse.	Unaffected.	Pleural effusion in 8 to 10 per cent. Mediastinal lymph node enlargement uncommon.	Diffuse disease occurs more often in a mixed pattern. (*See* page 1414.)
Hematogenous metastases.	Widespread.	Unaffected.	——	A rare manifestation of hematogenous metastases. (*See* page 1625.)
THROMBOEMBOLIC				
Fat embolism.	Diffuse, although predominantly peripheral.	Unaffected.	Fracture of extremities, pelvis, or axial skeleton usually present. Heart size normal.	Lesions appear within 1 to 2 days after trauma and resolve within 1 to 4 weeks. Opacities tend to be peripheral rather than central. Absence of cardiac enlargement and of signs of postcapillary hypertension aid in differentiation from pulmonary edema of cardiac origin. (*See* page 1782.)
Amniotic fluid embolism.	Generalized.	Unaffected.	If vascular occlusion is severe enough, the heart may be enlarged as a result of cor pulmonale.	Airspace pulmonary edema indistinguishable from that of any other cause. (*See* page 1788.)
CARDIOVASCULAR				
Pulmonary edema, either hydrostatic or permeability in type.	Usually bilateral and symmetric. Cortex of lung may be relatively spared (the "butterfly" pattern).	Commonly reduced.	Associated findings depend largely on the etiology of the edema — for example, signs of interstitial pulmonary edema (septal lines, and so forth) in edema of cardiac origin.	(*See* pages 1899 and 1927.)

Table continued on following page

Etiology	Anatomic Distribution	Volume of Thorax	Additional Findings	Comments
INHALATIONAL				
Acute aspiration pulmonary edema (near-drowning).	Diffuse.	Unaffected.	To be noted are the normal cardiac size and the absence of signs of pulmonary venous hypertension.	Roentgenographic pattern is one of diffuse patchy airspace consolidation typical of pulmonary edema. May occur with aspiration of fresh or sea water (in near-drowning), ethyl alcohol, kerosene, and, by far the most common, acid gastric juice (Mendelson's syndrome). (*See* pages 2387 and 2406.)
Acute berylliosis (fulminating variety).	Diffuse.	Unaffected.	———	Morphologic changes consist of severe proteinaceous edema of the lungs. Roentgenologic changes characteristically develop rapidly following an overwhelming exposure. (*See* page 2363.)
Acute berylliosis (insidious variety).	Diffuse.	Unaffected.	None.	Roentgenographic changes consist of diffuse bilateral "haziness" with subsequent development of irregular patchy densities scattered widely throughout the lungs; develop 1 to 4 weeks after the onset of symptoms. Roentgenographic clearing may take two to three months. (*See* page 2363.)

68

Acute silicoproteinosis.	Diffuse.	May be severely reduced.	Hilar lymph node enlargement.	Roentgenographic pattern is similar or identical to that of alveolar proteinosis. An acute, rapidly progressive course is characteristic. Most commonly seen in sandblasters. (*See* page 2300.)

DRUGS AND POISONS

Drugs

Acetylsalicylic acid (aspirin).	Diffuse.	Unaffected.	None.	Permeability pulmonary edema, usually following ingestion of large doses. (*See* page 2442.)
Heroin and other narcotics.	Diffuse.	Unaffected.	None.	Permeability pulmonary edema. Resolution often occurs in as brief a time as 24 to 48 hours. (*See* page 2444.)
Contrast media.	Diffuse.	Unaffected.	None.	Permeability pulmonary edema. Responsible media include ethiodized oil and high osmolar water-soluble agents. (*See* page 2444.)

Poisons (ingested or inhaled)

Fluorocarbon/hydrocarbon ingestion.	Bilateral and predominantly basal.	Unaffected.	A pneumatocele can develop occasionally as a consequence of bronchiolar obstruction.	The roentgenographic pattern consists of patchy airspace consolidation caused by edema. The hila tend to be hazy and indistinct. (*See* page 2451.)
Paraquat ingestion.	Predominantly lower zones early, then diffuse.	Unaffected.	None.	Roentgenographic changes appear 3 to 7 days after ingestion and consist initially of fine granular opacities, predominantly basal in location. This is followed shortly by a pattern of diffuse pulmonary edema. (*See* page 2448.)

Table continued on following page

Etiology	Anatomic Distribution	Volume of Thorax	Additional Findings	Comments
DRUGS AND POISONS *(Continued)* **Inhaled toxic gases and aerosols** Nitrogen dioxide. Sulfur dioxide. Hydrogen sulfide. Ammonia. Chlorine. Phosgene. Cadmium. Associated with burns.	Diffuse.	Unaffected.	None.	Acute pulmonary edema develops within hours of exposure, and usually clears completely if the patient survives. (*See* pages 2453 to 2464.)
METABOLIC Alveolar proteinosis.	Bilateral and symmetric, commonly in a "butterfly" distribution. Resolution tends to occur asymmetrically.	Unaffected.	None.	Differentiated from pulmonary edema on the basis of absence of cardiac enlargement and of signs of pulmonary venous hypertension; Kerley B lines have been reported, however. (*See* page 2572.)
IDIOPATHIC Sarcoidosis.	Diffuse.	Unaffected.	Hilar and mediastinal lymph node enlargement in many cases.	An uncommon pattern in this disease. May be the predominant pattern (in 20 per cent of patients) or associated with a reticulonodular pattern elsewhere in the lungs. (*See* page 2611.)

TABLE 10

**Diffuse Pulmonary Disease With a Predominantly
Nodular, Reticular, or Reticulonodular Pattern**

The large number of diseases capable of producing an "interstitial" pattern within the lungs has made this table the longest in the group. As with diseases characterized by an acinar pattern, "diffuse" involvement connotes affection of all lobes of both lungs, although the pattern may be more marked in some areas. Other abnormalities may be present, such as pleural effusion, hilar and mediastinal lymph node enlargement, and cardiac enlargement. The individual patterns may be described as follows.

NODULAR. The purely nodular interstitial diseases of the lungs perhaps are best epitomized by hematogenous infections such as miliary tuberculosis. Since the infecting organism arrives via the circulation and is trapped in the capillary sieve, it must be purely interstitial in location, at least early in its course. The pattern consists of discrete punctate opacities that range from tiny nodules 1 mm in diameter (barely visible roentgenographically) to 5 mm.

RETICULAR. This pattern consists of a network of linear opacities which may be regarded as a series of "rings" surrounding spaces of air density. It is useful to describe a reticular pattern according to the size of the "mesh": the terms fine, medium, and coarse are widely used and appear generally acceptable.

RETICULONODULAR. This pattern may be produced by a mixture of nodular deposits and diffuse linear thickening throughout the interstitial space. In addition, although a linear network throughout the interstitial tissue may appear roentgenographically as a purely reticular pattern, the orientation of some of the linear densities parallel to the x-ray beam may suggest a nodular component.

THE HONEYCOMB PATTERN. In this book, the term "honeycomb pattern" is restricted to a very coarse reticulation in which the airspaces in the "mesh" measure not less than 5 mm in diameter.

71

TABLE 10
Diffuse Pulmonary Disease With a Predominantly Nodular, Reticular, or Reticulonodular Pattern

Etiology	Anatomic Distribution	Volume of Thorax	Additional Findings	Comments
INFECTIOUS				
Bacteria				
Mycobacterium tuberculosis.	Generalized, uniform.	Unaffected.	None.	Characteristic miliary pattern resulting from hematogenous dissemination. (*See* page 919.)
Staphylococcus aureus.	Generalized, uniform.	Unaffected.	When of sufficient size, lesions may excavate to produce microabscesses.	Miliary pattern (hematogenous dissemination). (*See* page 836.)
Salmonella species.	Generalized, uniform.	Unaffected.	There may be disseminated destructive lesions of bone.	Miliary pattern (hematogenous dissemination). (*See* page 850.)
Fungi				
Coccidioides immitis.	Generalized, uniform.	Unaffected.	Generalized, hematogenous spread may lead to destructive lesions of bone.	Miliary pattern (hematogenous dissemination). (*See* page 965.)
Cryptococcus neoformans.	Generalized, uniform.	Unaffected.	None.	Miliary pattern (hematogenous dissemination). (*See* page 977.)
Paracoccidioides (Blastomyces) brasiliensis.	Generalized, uniform.	Unaffected.	None.	Hematogenous dissemination with production of miliary pattern is the only pulmonary manifestation of the disease. Seen only in South America. (*See* page 975.)

Blastomyces dermatitidis.	Generalized, uniform.	Unaffected.	Thoracic or remote bone involvement.	Miliary pattern (hematogenous dissemination). (*See* page 970.)
Histeplasma capsulatum.	Generalized, uniform.	Unaffected.	Hilar node enlargement in the majority of cases.	The "epidemic" form of the disease, typically developing in groups of people heavily exposed to organisms in caves or in locales of contaminated soil. Acute nodular opacities measuring 3 to 4 mm may heal to form multiple discrete calcifications many years later. (*See* page 947.)
Viruses				
Mycoplasma pneumoniae.	Generalized, uniform.	Unaffected.	Kerley B lines in some cases.	The presenting pattern in 28 of 100 cases in one series. Symptoms tend to be mild in contrast to the more common acute segmental disease. (*See* page 1038.)
Rubeola.	Generalized, uniform.	Unaffected.	Lymph node enlargement is common.	Reticulonodular. Primary measles infection of lungs may be associated with secondary bacterial pneumonia. (*See* page 1050.)
Cytomegalovirus.	Generalized, uniform.	Unaffected.	None.	Early stage manifestation, followed shortly by patchy acinar consolidation. (*See* page 1068.)
Parasites				
Schistosoma species (schistosomiasis).	Generalized, uniform.	Unaffected.	The central pulmonary arteries may be dilated secondary to vascular obstruction.	Hematogenous dissemination with production of a reticulonodular pattern. (*See* page 1111.)

73

Table continued on following page

Etiology	Anatomic Distribution	Volume of Thorax	Additional Findings	Comments
INFECTIOUS (Continued)				
Parasites (Continued)				
Filaria species (filariasis).	Generalized, uniform.	Unaffected.	Hilar lymph node enlargement in some cases.	Tropical pulmonary eosinophilia. Hematogenous dissemination with production of very fine reticulonodular pattern of low density. (*See* page 1097.)
Pneumocystis carinii.	Generalized, uniform.	Unaffected.	No lymph node enlargement or pleural effusion.	Early manifestation. (*See* page 1085.)
Toxoplasma gondii.	Generalized, uniform.	Unaffected.	Hilar lymph node enlargement common.	Represents the pattern seen in the early stages of diffuse disease. (*See* page 1081.)
IMMUNOLOGIC				
Idiopathic pulmonary hemorrhage and Goodpasture's syndrome.	Usually widespread but may be more prominent in the perihilar areas and the mid and lower lung zones.	May be a slight decrease in late stages of the disease.	———	Early in the disease, the pattern represents a transition stage from acute hemorrhage into the airspaces to complete resolution, but in the later stages interstitial fibrosis is permanent. (*See* page 1181.)
Progressive systemic sclerosis.	Generalized but more prominent in lung bases.	Serial roentgenographic studies may reveal progressive loss of lung volume.	Associated findings include esophageal dysperistalsis, terminal pulp calcinosis, absorption of distal phalanges, and widening of the periodontal membrane. Pleural effusion uncommon.	The roentgenographic pattern in the early stages consists of a fine reticulation which tends to coarsen and become reticulonodular as the disease progresses. Small cysts measuring up to 1 cm in diameter may be identified in the lung periphery, particularly in the bases. (*See* page 1220.)

74

Rheumatoid disease.	Generalized but more prominent in lung bases.	Serial roentgenographic studies may reveal progressive loss of lung volume.	Incidence of coexisting pleural effusion and pulmonary disease not clear, but the two are probably independent. Roentgenographic evidence of rheumatoid arthritis in most patients.	In the early stages the roentgenographic pattern is punctate or nodular in character; in the later or fibrotic stage the pattern consists of medium to coarse reticulation. (*See* page 1200.)
Extrinsic allergic alveolitis.	Generalized.	Unaffected.	Vary somewhat depending on specific causative antigen, chiefly regarding hilar and mediastinal lymph node enlargement.	Considerable similarity exists in the roentgenographic pattern observed with different antigens, ranging from a diffuse nodular pattern through coarse reticulation characteristic of diffuse interstitial fibrosis. While the pattern is generally "interstitial" in type, involvement of airspaces in the form of acinar opacities may be observed in most if not all during the acute stage of the disease. Irreversible changes of fibrosis tend to occur with continuous or repeated exposure. (*See* pages 1273 and 1286.)
Dermatomyositis and polymyositis.	Generalized but more prominent in lung bases.	Serial studies may reveal progressive loss of lung volume, particularly if polymyositis involves the muscles of respiration.	Additional findings may be those associated with progressive systemic sclerosis or rheumatoid disease. When polymyositis involves the muscles of respiration, small-volume lungs may be apparent.	In patients with diffuse lung involvement, the roentgenographic pattern is reticular or reticulonodular and may be indistinguishable from the changes of progressive systemic sclerosis or rheumatoid disease. These diseases sometimes occur in conjunction with primary malignancy elsewhere. (*See* page 1230.)
Sjögren's syndrome.	Generalized but more prominent in lung bases.	Unaffected.	This syndrome consists of a triad of keratoconjunctivitis sicca, xerostomia, and recurrent swelling of the parotid gland. Occasionally appears in association with any of the connective tissue diseases.	One third of patients show a diffuse reticulonodular pattern similar to that of other collagen diseases characterized by vascular involvement. Joint changes resemble rheumatoid or psoriatic arthritis. Remarkable female sex predominance. (*See* page 1233.)

Table continued on following page

TABLE 10
Diffuse Pulmonary Disease With a Predominantly Nodular, Reticular, or Reticulonodular Pattern (Continued)

Etiology	Anatomic Distribution	Volume of Thorax	Additional Findings	Comments
IMMUNOLOGIC *(Continued)* Systemic lupus erythematosus.	Generalized.	Serial studies may reveal progressive loss of lung volume.	Pleural effusions common. Enlargement of cardiovascular silhouette usually due to pericardial effusion.	Etiology of reticular pattern varied. (*See* page 1189.)
Necrotizing "sarcoidal" angiitis and granulomatosis.	Generalized.	Unaffected.	——	Predominantly nodular pattern. Nodules may be well-defined or ill-defined. Pattern indistinguishable from sarcoidosis roentgenologically but associated with angiitis and necrosis pathologically. (*See* page 1258.)
NEOPLASTIC Bronchiolo-alveolar carcinoma.	Diffuse.	Unaffected.	Pleural effusion in 8 to 10 per cent, always in association with pulmonary involvement.	The roentgenographic pattern is basically nodular; less common than a mixed pattern. Metastatic carcinoma of the pancreas may produce a pattern indistinguishable roentgenologically or morphologically. (*See* page 1414.)
Lymphangitic carcinomatosis.	Commonly generalized but more prominent in the lower lung zones.	Serial roentgenographic studies may reveal progressive reduction in volume.	Hilar or mediastinal lymph node enlargement is frequent but is not necessary to the diagnosis. Kerley B lines frequent.	Although the basic change is linear or reticular, there may be a coarse nodular component as well. (*See* page 1632.)
Hodgkin's disease.	Generalized.	Unaffected.	Mediastinal and hilar lymph node enlargement almost invariably associated.	Differentiation from sarcoidosis or lymphangitic carcinomatosis may be difficult or impossible on purely roentgenologic grounds. (*See* page 1507.)

Non-Hodgkin's lymphoma.	Diffuse.	Unaffected.	Pleural effusion in about one third of cases. Mediastinal and hilar lymph node enlargement may be inconspicuous or absent.	In some cases of large cell lymphoma, this diffuse pattern may be due to Sjögren's syndrome. The roentgenographic pattern may simulate lymphangitic carcinomatosis. (*See* page 1535.)
Leukemia.	Diffuse.	Unaffected.	Mediastinal and hilar lymph node enlargement may be present but not necessarily. Pleural effusion in some cases.	This is the usual pattern of pulmonary parenchymal involvement, but tends to occur only in the terminal stages of the disease. Resembles lymphangitic carcinomatosis. (*See* page 1554.)
Waldenström's macroglobulinemia.	Diffuse.	Unaffected.	Pleural effusion in about 50 per cent of cases.	This rare lymphoproliferative disorder is one of the plasma cell dyscrasias. (*See* page 1552.)
THROMBOEMBOLIC Embolism from oily contrast media.	Diffuse, uniform.	Unaffected.	None.	The typical pattern is finely reticular; complete clearing usually occurs within 48 to 72 hours, although an abnormal pattern may persist for up to 11 days. In the early stages an arborizing pattern may be apparent owing due to filling of arterioles with contrast medium (similar to that seen on pulmonary arteriography). This complication usually occurs following lymphangiography with ultrafluid Lipiodol. (*See* page 1803.)
Talc granulomatosis of drug addicts.	Usually generalized.	May be reduced in the presence of severe fibrosis.	Pulmonary arterial hypertension and cor pulmonale in advanced cases.	Creates a pure micronodular pattern similar to alveolar microlithiasis. (*See* page 1794.)

Table continued on following page

TABLE 10
Diffuse Pulmonary Disease With a Predominantly Nodular, Reticular, or Reticulonodular Pattern *(Continued)*

Etiology	Anatomic Distribution	Volume of Thorax	Additional Findings	Comments
THROMBOEMBOLIC *(Continued)* Metallic mercury embolism.	Predominantly lower lung zones.	Unaffected.	A local collection of mercury may be present in the heart, usually near the apex of the right ventricle.	Roentgenographic appearance distinctive because of the very high density of the intravascular mercury. May be in the form of spherules or of short tubular opacities. (*See* page 1803.)
Schistosomiasis.	Generalized.	Unaffected.	May be associated with signs of pulmonary arterial hypertension and cor pulmonale.	Presumably results from the passage of ova through vessel walls and the foreign body reaction to them. (*See* page 1111.)
CARDIOVASCULAR Interstitial pulmonary edema.	Diffuse but predominantly lower lung zones.	May be reduced.	Varies with the etiology of the edema, but usually those associated with pulmonary venous hypertension.	Roentgenographic pattern consists of loss of normal sharp definition of pulmonary vascular markings and thickening of the interlobular septa (Kerley B lines). (*See* page 1790.)
Pulmonary fibrosis secondary to chronic post-capillary hypertension.	Predominantly mid and lower lung zones.	Unaffected.	Typical cardiac configuration of chronic mitral valve disease. Almost invariably associated with signs of severe pulmonary venous and arterial hypertension. Ossific nodules may be present.	Roentgenographic pattern consists of a rather coarse but poorly defined reticulation. Probably related to recurrent episodes of airspace and interstitial edema and hemorrhage. (*See* page 1876.)
INHALATIONAL Silicosis (simple).	Generalized but often predominantly mid and upper lung zones.	Little affected.	Hilar lymph node enlargement frequent, uncommonly associated with "eggshell calcification" (5 per cent). Pleural thickening in late stages. Kerley A and B lines are common and may be present without visible nodules.	The roentgenographic pattern ranges from well-defined nodular opacities of uniform density ranging from 1 to 10 mm in diameter to a reticular or reticulonodular appearance. (*See* page 2289.)

78

Coal workers' pneumoconiosis (simple).	Generalized.	Unaffected.	Enlargement of hilar lymph nodes is present in some cases but is seldom a predominant feature.	The roentgenographic pattern is typically nodular but may be predominantly reticular in the early stages. Nodules range from 1 to 10 mm in size and tend to be somewhat less well defined than in silicosis. (*See* page 2313.)
Asbestosis.	In the early stages, predominantly lower lung zones; later generalized.	Normal or slightly reduced.	The pleural manifestations dominate the picture roentgenographically and consist of plaque formation and general thickening with or without calcification. Hilar lymph node enlargement is seldom if ever a notable feature.	The roentgenographic pattern may be divided into three stages: a fine reticulation occupying predominantly the lower lung zones and creating a ground-glass appearance of the lungs—the early changes; a stage in which the interstitial reticulation becomes more marked, producing the "shaggy heart" sign; and a late stage in which reticulation is generalized throughout the lungs. Note high incidence of associated neoplasia. (*See* page 2336.)
Talcosis.	Identical to asbestosis.	As with asbestosis.	The hallmark in the roentgenologic diagnosis of talcosis is pleural plaque formation — often diaphragmatic in position and massive. Large opacities may develop identical to those seen in silicosis and coal workers' pneumoconiosis.	Pulmonary involvement similar to asbestosis. (*See* page 2354.)
Kaolin (china-clay) pneumoconiosis.	Generalized.	Unaffected.	Progressive massive fibrosis may occur as a late manifestation, as in silicosis and coal workers' pneumoconiosis.	The roentgenographic pattern ranges from no more than a generalized increase in lung markings to a diffuse nodular or "miliary" mottling. (*See* page 2356.)

Table continued on following page

TABLE 10
Diffuse Pulmonary Disease With a Predominantly Nodular, Reticular, or Reticulonodular Pattern (Continued)

Etiology	Anatomic Distribution	Volume of Thorax	Additional Findings	Comments
INHALATIONAL (Continued) Chronic berylliosis.	Diffuse.	In advanced cases there may be marked loss of lung volume.	Focal areas of emphysema may be identified in advanced cases, usually in the upper lobes. Spontaneous pneumothorax occurs in over 10 per cent of patients.	The roentgenographic pattern varies with degree of exposure: if minor, there is a diffuse granular "haziness"; with moderate exposure, the pattern is nodular, the nodules being ill-defined and of moderate size (calcification of nodules has been observed); in advanced cases, the pattern may be chiefly reticular. (See page 2363.)
Aluminum pneumoconiosis (aluminosis, bauxitosis, Shaver's disease).	Diffuse.	Considerable loss of lung volume may occur.	Pleural thickening occasionally. Emphysematous bullae develop commonly and are associated with a high incidence of pneumothorax.	The roentgenographic pattern consists of a fine to coarse reticular pattern, sometimes with a nodular component. (See page 2366.)
Pneumoconiosis due to inert radiopaque dusts. Siderosis. Argyrosiderosis. Stannosis (tin oxide). Baritosis (barium sulfate). Antimony pneumoconiosis. Rare earth pneumoconiosis (cerium, etc.).	Generalized.	Unaffected.	Lymph node enlargement is not a feature.	In siderosis, the roentgenographic pattern is reticulonodular in type, the deposits being of rather low density compared with the silicotic nodule. In the siderosis of silver polishers, a fine stippled pattern is created. If the free silica content of dust is high (siderosilicosis), the pattern is indistinguishable from that of silicosis. The roentgenographic pattern of the other dusts is basically nodular, the nodules being of very high density. None of these dusts is fibrogenic. (See page 2357.)

80

Thesaurosis.	Diffuse.	Unaffected.	None.	A questionable entity. Pattern consists of a fine micronodulation which tends to clear with discontinuance of exposure to hair spray. (*See* page 2467.)

AIRWAYS DISEASE

Chronic obstructive pulmonary disease (chronic bronchitic type).	Generalized, uniform.	Slight to moderate increase.	Signs of pulmonary arterial hypertension are inevitable, often associated with cor pulmonale.	The pattern is better described as a coarse increase in lung markings rather than reticular or reticulonodular. May be referred to as "increased markings (IM)" emphysema. (*See* page 2135.)
Cystic fibrosis.	Generalized, uniform.	Considerable overinflation.	May be associated with segmental areas of consolidation or atelectasis due to bronchopneumonia or bronchiectasis.	The pattern is one of accentuation of the linear markings throughout the lungs giving a coarse reticular appearance. (*See* page 2208.)
Diffuse panbronchiolitis.	Generalized but predominantly lower lobes.	Overinflation, characteristically severe and generalized.	Large cystic spaces may be evident on CT.	Unique to Japan. A nodular pattern is characteristic as is hyperinflation. (*See* page 2224.)
Familial dysautonomia (Riley-Day syndrome).	Generalized.	Increased.	Local areas of segmental consolidation and atelectasis may be present, particularly in the right upper lobe and less frequently the right middle and left lower lobes.	The roentgenographic pattern is identical to that of cystic fibrosis. (*See* page 2219.)

DRUGS AND POISONS
Drug-induced

Nitrofurantoin.	Generalized.	Unaffected.	Pleural effusion in some cases.	Disease occurs in two forms, acute and chronic. In both, the pattern consists of a diffuse reticulation. The acute form is invariably associated with peripheral blood eosinophilia, the chronic form sometimes. (*See* page 2434.)

Table continued on following page

TABLE 10
Diffuse Pulmonary Disease With a Predominantly Nodular, Reticular, or Reticulonodular Pattern *(Continued)*

Etiology	Anatomic Distribution	Volume of Thorax	Additional Findings	Comments
DRUGS AND POISONS *(Continued)* **Drug-induced** *(Continued)* Busulfan. Bleomycin. Mitomycin. Pepleomycin. Cyclophosphamide. Chlorambucil. Melphalan. BCNU. Amiodarone. Phenytoin.	Generalized.	Unaffected.	None.	Each of these drugs causes a diffuse reticulonodular pattern initially; this may progress to patchy airspace disease. *(See pages 2418 to 2438. See also Table 14–1, page 2419.)*
METABOLIC Lipid storage disease Gaucher's disease. Niemann-Pick disease. Hermansky-Pudlak syndrome.	Generalized.	Unaffected.	Occasionally lytic bone lesions in Gaucher's disease.	Pattern is usually reticulonodular but may be miliary. *(See pages 2590 to 2592.)*
Bronchopulmonary amyloidosis.	Generalized.	Unaffected.	Hilar and mediastinal lymph node enlargement may be massive, and nodes can be densely calcified.	This is the diffuse alveolar septal form of the disease. *(See page 2578.)*

82

IDIOPATHIC

Sarcoidosis.	Usually generalized but in stages of development or resolution may show some lack of uniformity.	Usually unaffected although fibrosis may be associated with emphysema and overinflation.	Hilar and mediastinal lymph node enlargement often constitutes the earliest roentgenologic finding, with diffuse lung involvement developing subsequently (with or without disappearance of the node enlargement). In approximately 25 per cent of cases, the pulmonary changes exist alone.	The pattern is usually reticulonodular in type, although ranging from purely nodular to purely reticular. In the approximately 20 per cent of cases that progress to fibrosis the pattern is coarsely reticular, somewhat uneven in distribution and associated with bulla formation and generalized overinflation. (*See* page 2611.)
Cryptogenic fibrosing alveolitis; interstitial pulmonary fibrosis.	There is a predilection for the lower lung zones in the early stages, but becoming more generalized and uniform as the disease progresses.	Sequential studies will show progressive loss of lung volume.	Hilar lymph node enlargement and pleural effusion do not occur.	In the early stages the pattern is one of fine reticulation predominantly in the lung bases; the later stage is characterized by a generalized coarse reticular or reticulonodular pattern with "honeycombing" in some cases. (*See* page 2662.)
Eosinophilic granuloma.	Diffuse but with a tendency for predominance of lesions in the upper lung zones.	Usually normal or increased.	Hilar and mediastinal lymph-node enlargement are exceedingly rare as is pleural effusion. Spontaneous pneumothorax in some cases.	The roentgenographic pattern varies with the stage of the disease, beginning with nodular and progressing to reticulonodular and finally to a typical honeycomb pattern. Probably the most common cause of a honeycomb pattern.
Pulmonary lymphangioleio-myomatosis and tuberous sclerosis.	Usually generalized but predominantly basal.	Increased.	Chylous pleural effusion and pneumothorax common. Sclerotic (and sometimes lytic) lesions in bone.	The basic pattern is coarse reticulonodular in type and may progress to a typical "honeycomb" appearance. (*See* page 2672.)

83

Table continued on following page

TABLE 10
Diffuse Pulmonary Disease With a Predominantly Nodular, Reticular, or Reticulonodular Pattern *(Continued)*

Etiology	Anatomic Distribution	Volume of Thorax	Additional Findings	Comments
IDIOPATHIC *(Continued)*				
Neurofibromatosis.	Generalized.	May be increased.	Diffuse interstitial fibrosis usually associated with multiple bullae. Scoliosis and mediastinal neurofibromas.	Fibrosis is widespread with some basal predominance, whereas bullae are predominantly upper zonal. *(See* page 2679.)
Alveolar microlithiasis.	Diffuse.	Unaffected.	Spontaneous pneumothorax is a rare complication.	The roentgenographic pattern is virtually pathognomonic, consisting of a myriad of tiny micronodular opacities. Conceivably could be confused with similar (although less numerous) opacities in talcosis of intravenous drug abuse. *(See* page 2693.)
OTHER CAUSES Spider angiomas in cirrhosis of the liver.	Predominantly basal.	Unaffected.	None.	Pattern consists of ill-defined nodules of small size. Associated with hypoxemia due to veno-arterial shunting. *(See* page 2999.)

84

TABLE 11

Diffuse Pulmonary Disease
With a Mixed Acinar and Reticulonodular Pattern

The pattern created by combined airspace consolidation and interstitial disease is best exemplified by pulmonary edema secondary to pulmonary venous hypertension. The roentgenographic manifestations of interstitial involvement consist of increased size and loss of definition of lung markings due to the presence of edema fluid within the bronchovascular sheath; airspace consolidation is manifested by discrete and confluent "fluffy" opacities characteristic of acinar-filling processes.

Another example of the mixed pattern is that produced by generalized bronchiolo-alveolar carcinoma: nodular and acinar components reflect the replacement of air spaces by malignant cells, and the linear or reticular component is due to the extension of carcinoma along the bronchovascular bundles, both within and around lymphatics (lymphangitic carcinoma).

TABLE 11
Diffuse Pulmonary Disease With a Mixed Acinar and Reticulonodular Pattern

Etiology	Anatomic Distribution	Volume of Thorax	Additional Findings	Comments
INFECTIOUS				
Cytomegalovirus.	Generalized, uniform.	Usually unaffected.	None.	Combined interstitial and airspace disease with production of mixed reticulonodular and acinar patterns. (*See* page 1068.)
Pneumocystis carinii.	Usually generalized.	Unaffected.	None.	Pattern is combined reticulonodular and acinar. Sometimes occurs in combination with cytomegalovirus infection. (*See* page 1085.)
Mycoplasma pneumoniae and all viruses listed in Table 4.	Generalized, uniform.	Unaffected or slightly decreased.	None.	Diffuse reticular pattern early, with superimposition of patchy airspace consolidation. (*See* page 1036.)
Strongyloides stercoralis.	Generalized.	Unaffected.	None.	Represents overwhelming infestation in a compromised host. (*See* page 1094.)
IMMUNOLOGIC				
Idiopathic pulmonary hemorrhage and Goodpasture's syndrome.	Usually widespread but may be more prominent in the perihilar areas and the mid and lower lung zones.	Usually unaffected.	Rarely hilar lymph node enlargement. Coalescence of lesions may permit visualization of an air bronchogram.	The mixed pattern is caused by a combination of patchy airspace consolidation from hemorrhage and the presence of hemosiderin and fibrous tissue in the interstitium. It may clear completely or may leave a residuum of reticulation due to irreversible interstitial fibrosis. (*See* page 1181.)

Extrinsic allergic alveolitis.	Generalized.	Unaffected.	Vary somewhat, depending on specific causative antigen, chiefly regarding hilar and mediastinal lymph node enlargement.	The majority of these cases are manifested by a relatively pure "interstitial" pattern which is either nodular or reticulonodular. However, in some cases acinar shadows representing airspace involvement are superimposed on the reticular pattern during the acute stage of the disease. (*See* page 1273.)
NEOPLASTIC Bronchiolo-alveolar carcinoma.	Generalized.	Unaffected.	Prominent linear opacities extending along the bronchovascular bundles toward the hila usually represent lymphatic permeation. Pleural effusion in 8 to 10 per cent. Mediastinal lymph node enlargement uncommon.	The mixed pattern consists of acinar, nodular, and reticulonodular components. (*See* page 1414.)
CARDIOVASCULAR Pulmonary edema.	Usually generalized.	May be reduced.	Cardiomegaly common but not invariable.	Combined interstitial and airspace edema. (*See* page 1899.)
DRUGS AND POISONS Bleomycin.	Diffuse.	Unaffected.	None.	Toxicity in 1 to 2 per cent caused by oxidants in most cases, hypersensitivity in a minority. As with other drugs in this column, the roentgenographic pattern is reticulonodular at the beginning, then becomes acinar. (*See* page 2418.)
Methotrexate.⎫ Azathioprine.⎭	Diffuse.	Unaffected.	Rarely enlargement of hilar lymph nodes.	Toxicity in 5 per cent of patients caused by a cellular immune response. Mortality rate about 1 per cent. (*See* page 2433.)
Busulfan.	Diffuse.	Unaffected.	Pleural effusion very uncommon.	Clinically recognized toxicity occurs in only about 4 per cent of patients and only with long-term use. (*See* page 2427.)

Table continued on following page

TABLE 11
Diffuse Pulmonary Disease With a Mixed Acinar and Reticulonodular Pattern *(Continued)*

Etiology	Anatomic Distribution	Volume of Thorax	Additional Findings	Comments
DRUGS AND POISONS *(Continued)*				
Mitomycin.	Lower zonal predominance.	Unaffected.	Pleural effusion is a more common feature than in other cytotoxic drug reactions.	Mortality rate is said to be about 50 per cent. (*See* page 2426.)
Cyclophosphamide.	Diffuse.	Can be reduced in children.	Occasionally, severe airspace pulmonary edema.	Incidence of toxicity very low, probably less than 1 per cent. (*See* page 2428.)
Amiodarone.	Diffuse with some lower zonal predominance.	Unaffected.	Sometimes accompanied by peripheral consolidation resembling chronic eosinophilic pneumonia.	Incidence of toxicity ranges from 1 to 6 per cent. (*See* page 2438.)
Gold.	Diffuse.	Unaffected.	None.	The mechanism is thought to be a hypersensitivity reaction, approximately one third of patients showing peripheral eosinophilia. (*See* page 2443.)
IDIOPATHIC				
Sarcoidosis.	Generalized.	Unaffected.	Hilar and mediastinal lymph node enlargement may coexist.	A mixed acinar and reticulonodular pattern is more common than a predominantly acinar pattern alone. (*See* page 2611.)
Diffuse fibrosing alveolitis (desquamative interstitial pneumonitis).	Generalized but with lower zone predominance	Progressive loss of lung volume common.	Hilar and mediastinal lymph node enlargement uncommon.	Early changes have been described as "ground-glass" opacification of both lungs. (*See* page 2662.)

TABLE 12

Generalized Pulmonary Oligemia

This table includes all diseases in which there is reduction in the caliber of the pulmonary arterial tree throughout the lungs. As stressed previously, appreciation of such vascular change is a subjective process based on a thorough familiarity with the normal. Since reduction in the size of peripheral vessels constitutes the main criterion of diagnosis of all diseases in this category, differentiation depends upon secondary signs. The two ancillary signs of major importance are abnormal size and configuration of the central hilar vessels and general pulmonary overinflation. Three combinations of changes are possible:

1. Small peripheral vessels; no overinflation; normal or small hila. This combination indicates reduction in pulmonary blood flow from central causes and is virtually pathognomonic of cardiac disease, usually congenital.

2. Small peripheral vessels; no overinflation; enlarged hilar pulmonary arteries. This combination may result from peripheral or central causes (respectively, primary pulmonary arterial hypertension or massive pulmonary artery thrombosis without infarction).

3. Small peripheral vessels; general pulmonary overinflation; normal or enlarged hilar pulmonary arteries. This combination is virtually pathognomonic of pulmonary emphysema.

TABLE 12
Generalized Pulmonary Oligemia

Etiology	Differential Characteristics	Comments
DEVELOPMENTAL Pulmonary artery stenosis or coarctation.	Absence of overinflation and expiratory air trapping differentiates this from emphysema. Pulmonary arteriography essential to differentiate it from primary pulmonary hypertension or multiple peripheral embolization.	Diffuse pulmonary oligemia occurs when lesions are *multiple* and *peripheral*. Pulmonary arterial hypertension and cor pulmonale common. Associated cardiovascular anomalies frequent (60 per cent), particularly pulmonic stenosis. (*See* page 735.)

Congenital cardiac anomalies
  Isolated pulmonic stenosis.
  Tetralogy of Fallot with pulmonary atresia.
  Persistent truncus arteriosus (type IV).
  Ebstein's anomaly.
	Cardiac enlargement present in some cases; no overinflation or air trapping. Hila diminutive as a rule, permitting differentiation from primary pulmonary hypertension and multiple peripheral embolization (exception is poststenotic dilatation of main or left pulmonary artery in valvular pulmonic stenosis).	Pulmonary vascular pattern formed partly or wholly by hypertrophied bronchial circulation (may be studied by selective bronchial arteriography or flood aortography). (*See* page 755.)

INFECTIOUS *Schistosoma* species.	Indistinguishable from pattern of primary pulmonary hypertension. Central pulmonary arteries can be huge. Absence of overinflation.	More common method of presentation is a diffuse reticulonodular pattern. (*See* page 1111.)

IMMUNOLOGIC

Pulmonary hypertension associated with connective tissue disease, notably SLE, progressive systemic sclerosis, and the CREST syndrome.	Indistinguishable from primary pulmonary hypertension. No overinflation.	Often associated with Raynaud's phenomenon. (*See* page 1230.)

NEOPLASTIC

Metastases from trophoblastic neoplasms.	Indistinguishable from primary pulmonary hypertension. No overinflation.	Acute cor pulmonale responds to treatment in some cases. (*See* page 1651.)

THROMBOEMBOLIC

Widespread embolic disease to small arteries.	Indistinguishable from primary pulmonary hypertension. No overinflation.	Multiple pulmonary emboli result in pulmonary artery hypertension; in contrast to emphysema, lung volume is either normal or decreased. (*See* pages 1718 and 1848.)

CARDIOVASCULAR

Chronic postcapillary hypertension (mitral stenosis).	Characteristic configuration of enlarged heart, particularly left atrium. Diffuse oligemia represents late stage of chronic venous and arterial hypertension.	Commonly associated with episodes of interstitial or airspace edema. Roentgenographic evidence of hemosiderosis and ossific nodules in an occasional case. (*See* page 1861.)
Primary pulmonary hypertension.	Main and hilar pulmonary arteries are enlarged and show increased amplitude of pulsation fluoroscopically. Peripheral vessels diminutive. Absence of overinflation.	Preponderance in young women; familial tendency; dramatic response to intravenous injection of acetylcholine in some cases. (*See* page 1842.)

Table continued on following page

TABLE 12
Generalized Pulmonary Oligemia *(Continued)*

Etiology	Differential Characteristics	Comments
AIRWAYS DISEASE		
Emphysema.	Generalized overinflation serves to differentiate this disease from others characterized by diffuse oligemia. Bullae may be present.	The oligemia may be predominant in the upper or lower lung zones or in one lung. *(See* page 2120.)
Bullous disease of the lung.	Margins of bullae may be identified as curved, hairline opacities. Hyperinflation as in diffuse emphysema.	A pattern of diffuse oligemia is rare in bullous disease of the lungs without emphysema, but may be seen when bullae are numerous and have enlarged maximally. *(See* page 2166.)

TABLE 13

Unilateral, Lobar, or Segmental Pulmonary Oligemia

The same three combinations of changes apply in this pattern as in general pulmonary oligemia (the major difference between local and general oligemia is in its effect on pulmonary hemodynamics):

1. Small peripheral vessels, no overinflation; normal or small hilum. This is epitomized by lobar or unilateral hyperlucent lung (Swyer-James or Macleod's syndrome).

2. Small peripheral vessels; no overinflation; enlarged hilar pulmonary arteries (or an enlarged hilum). This combination is due almost invariably to unilateral pulmonary artery embolism without infarction.

3. Small peripheral vessels; overinflation; normal hilar pulmonary arteries. This combination is distinctive of obstructive emphysema.

TABLE 13
Unilateral, Lobar, or Segmental Pulmonary Oligemia

Etiology	Differential Characteristics	Comments
DEVELOPMENTAL		
Hypogenetic lung syndrome.	Anomalous vein forms "scimitar sign," which is diagnostic.	Partial hypoplasia of the right lung and right pulmonary artery; associated anomalies include dextrocardia, mirror-image bronchial tree, and anomalous venous drainage of right lung to inferior vena cava. Right lung supplied by systemic arteries, in part or wholly (*see* page 748.)
Proximal interruption of the right or left pulmonary artery.	Absent or diminutive hilum. Differentiation from Swyer-James (Macleod's) syndrome by absence of air trapping on forced expiration. Confirmation of diagnosis by pulmonary arteriography.	Involved lung hypoplastic and of reduced volume; supplied by hypertrophied bronchial circulation. Anomalous artery usually on side opposite aortic arch: when on *left,* high incidence of associated cardiovascular anomalies. (*See* page 729.)
Anomalous origin of left pulmonary artery from the right.	If right main bronchus is compressed, whole right lung may be radiolucent due to air trapping — thus, lung is *overinflated.* Confirmation by demonstration of posterior displacement of barium-filled esophagus due to interposition of anomalous artery between lower trachea and esophagus: arteriography diagnostic.	If anomalous artery compresses trachea rather than right main bronchus, both lungs will show overinflation and expiratory air trapping. Severe compression may result in atelectasis of right lung. (*See* page 731.)

Congenital bronchial atresia.	Almost invariably associated with a smooth, lobulated soft tissue mass (due to inspissated mucus) distal to the point of atresia.	May involve a variety of segmental bronchi but most commonly affects the apicoposterior segment of the left upper lobe. Affected bronchopulmonary segments are air-containing owing to collateral air drift. (*See* page 721.)
Neonatal lobar hyperinflation (congenital lobar emphysema).	Characterized by severe overinflation of a pulmonary lobe, most commonly the left upper or right middle lobe. Air trapping is severe and results in marked enlargement of the lobe and contralateral displacement of the mediastinum.	Only about a third of cases become manifest at birth, the remainder not being recognized until some weeks later. Cyanosis may develop in severe cases. (*See* page 722.)
INFECTIOUS		
Mycobacterium tuberculosis (primary).	Ipsilateral hilar lymph node enlargement is present in most cases of primary tuberculosis. There is a predilection for anterior segment of upper lobe and medial segment of middle lobe.	Overinflation and oligemia result from partial bronchial obstruction. Although the majority of cases with this pattern are consequent upon extrabronchial compression from lymph nodes, some may develop as a result of bronchostenosis from tuberculous granuloma. Atelectasis may replace localized oligemia at a later stage. (*See* page 895.)
Staphylococcus aureus.	Large pneumatoceles develop as a complication of acute staphylococcal pneumonia and may fill an entire hemithorax. Air-fluid levels are present in some cases. Characteristically undergo rapid change in size.	Common in infants and children, rare in adults. (*See* page 836.)
IMMUNOLOGIC		
Relapsing polychondritis.	Oligemia is usually unilateral and involves a whole lung. It results from hypoxic vasoconstriction secondary to alveolar hypoventilation caused by narrowing of a major bronchus. Air trapping is present on expiration.	A rare cause of local oligemia. (*See* page 1238.)

Table continued on following page

TABLE 13
Unilateral, Lobar, or Segmental Pulmonary Oligemia *(Continued)*

Etiology	Differential Characteristics	Comments
NEOPLASTIC		
Pulmonary carcinoma.	A segment, lobe, or whole lung may be affected. A mass is almost invariably identifiable. Air trapping may be noted on forced expiration.	This is a rare manifestation of pulmonary carcinoma. It may progress to a pattern of homogeneous segmental consolidation and atelectasis as a result of obstructive pneumonitis. Lymphatic spread of neoplasm to hilar lymph nodes occasionally results in compression of a bronchus, with resultant oligemia. (*See* page 1369.)
Carcinoid tumor.	Air trapping on expiration and oligemia may be followed by atelectasis or obstructive pneumonitis.	Volume of affected parenchyma usually smaller than normal at full inspiration. Air trapping and oligemia result from partial endobronchial obstruction and hypoxic vasoconstriction. (*See* pages 1477, 1497, and 1577.)
Tracheobronchial gland tumors.		
All neoplasms of soft tissues, bone, and cartilage listed in Table 2.		
Hodgkin's disease.	Asymmetric lymph node enlargement in paratracheal, retrosternal, and hilar areas is almost invariable.	Local oligemia is a rare manifestation of endobronchial Hodgkin's disease. (*See* page 1507.)
Non-Hodgkin's lymphoma.	Usually in association with hilar and mediastinal lymph node enlargement. Indistinguishable from Hodgkin's disease.	A rare manifestation of the secondary form of non-Hodgkin's lymphoma; results from partial endobronchial obstruction. (*See* page 1535.)

THROMBOEMBOLIC

Pulmonary thromboembolism without infarction.

Almost invariably associated with obstruction of a major pulmonary artery (*e.g.,* lobar). Affected artery is characteristically widened and of sharper than normal definition. The involved bronchopulmonary segments may show moderate loss of volume – of value in differentiation from other causes of local oligemia.

Local oligemia resulting from thromboembolism constitutes Westermark's sign. (*See* page 1718.)

INHALATIONAL

Foreign body aspiration.

Lower lobe predominance, invariably segmental in distribution. Foreign body identifiable as an opaque shadow in some cases.

Air trapping and local oligemia are more common manifestations of foreign body inhalation than atelectasis or obstructive pneumonitis. (*See* page 2382.)

AIRWAYS DISEASE

Local obstructive emphysema.

In addition to showing air trapping on expiration (as in Swyer-James syndrome), affected zones are overinflated at TLC.

Approximately 50 per cent of cases of emphysema have local rather than diffuse involvement of the lungs as assessed roentgenologically, although function tests usually indicate generalized disease. Affected areas may be upper zones or lower zones, more frequently the latter. (*See* page 2120.)

Unilateral or lobar emphysema (Swyer-James syndrome).

Oligemia characteristically involves a whole lung, producing unilateral radiolucency; however, single lobes may be similarly affected. Both the hilar and peripheral vessels are diminutive, although structurally normal. The volume of affected lung at TLC is normal or reduced, seldom if ever increased. Air trapping on expiration is a *sine qua non* to the diagnosis, and permits differentiation from agenesis of a pulmonary artery. Bronchiectasis is demonstrable in most cases.

There is convincing evidence that this abnormality results from acute pneumonia during infancy or childhood, frequently of viral etiology; infection of the peripheral airways leads to bronchiolitis obliterans and a morphologic picture virtually indistinguishable from emphysema. (*See* page 2177.)

97

Table continued on following page

TABLE 13
Unilateral, Lobar, or Segmental Pulmonary Oligemia *(Continued)*

Etiology	Differential Characteristics	Comments
AIRWAYS DISEASE *(Continued)* Bullae.	Characterized by sharply defined, air-containing spaces bounded by curvilinear, hairline shadows; range in size from 1 cm to the volume of a hemithorax. Vascular markings are absent; adjacent lung parenchyma is compressed. Overinflation and air trapping are usual.	Predominantly unilateral in contrast to the bilateral disease described in Table 12. Unlike unilateral emphysema, the vasculature is absent rather than attenuated. (*See* pages 2132 and 2166.)
METABOLIC Bronchopulmonary amyloidosis.	A manifestation of endobronchial amyloid deposits producing partial bronchial obstruction. Parenchymal lesions may be present as well.	A rare cause of local oligemia. This is the tracheobronchial form of this disorder. (*See* page 2578.)
IDIOPATHIC Sarcoidosis.	Oligemia results from partial bronchial obstruction and consequent air trapping and overinflation. Usually lobar or multilobar. Diagnosis may be suspected from symmetric hilar and paratracheal lymph node enlargement.	A rare cause of local oligemia. Although bronchial compression from enlarged nodes may be the cause, obstruction more often results from endobronchial sarcoid deposits. (*See* page 2611.)
Neurofibromatosis.	Multiple bullae, usually with upper zonal predominance, often associated with diffuse interstitial fibrosis but can occur alone.	Usually associated with numerous cutaneous nodules and other stigmata. (*See* page 2679.)

TABLE 14

Pleural Effusion Unassociated With Other
Roentgenographic Evidence of Disease in the Thorax

This title is self-explanatory. Effusion may be unilateral or bilateral. It must be emphasized that the lack of association with other abnormalities in the chest implies the absence of other *roentgenologically demonstrable* abnormality. Obviously, disease may be present but be roentgenographically invisible; for example, pulmonary involvement in rheumatoid disease may have no definite roentgenographic manifestations, although a considerable degree of pulmonary interstitial fibrosis may be apparent histologically. Conversely, diseases in which pulmonary abnormality is obscured by an effusion (e.g., lobar collapse due to an obstructing endobronchial cancer) are *not* included in this table, since the presence of underlying pulmonary disease would be clearly demonstrable by CT or after thoracentesis.

TABLE 14
Pleural Effusion Unassociated With Other Roentgenographic Evidence of Disease in the Thorax

Etiology	Character of the Fluid	Criteria for Presumptive Diagnosis	Criteria for Positive Diagnosis	Comments
INFECTIOUS				
Bacteria				
Mycobacterium tuberculosis.	Serous exudate. Predominantly lymphocytic reaction; erythrocytes may be present but seldom in great numbers. Blood glucose levels below 25 mg/100 ml highly suggestive (N.B.: differentiate from effusions of rheumatoid disease).	Combination of positive tuberculin reaction and predominantly lymphocytic pleural fluid.	Positive pleural biopsy. Culture of tubercle bacili from pleural fluid.	A negative tuberculin test may be found in early cases. Strong tendency to subsequent development of active pulmonary tuberculosis if effusion not treated. Effusions rarely bilateral. A manifestation of primary tuberculosis more common in the adult (approximately 40 per cent) than in children (10 per cent). (*See* page 2717.)
Viruses				
All viruses and *Mycoplasma.*	Serous exudate.	None.	Elevated agglutinin titer to offending organism.	May be bilateral. (*See* page 2722.)
Subphrenic abscess.	Serous exudate.	Elevation and fixation of hemidiaphragm.	Gas and fluid in subphrenic space.	More commonly associated with basal pulmonary disease ("plate" atelectasis or pneumonitis). (*See* page 2736.)

IMMUNOLOGIC

Systemic lupus erythematosus.	Serous exudate.	Clinical findings of typical rash, renal disease, heart murmur, and so forth.	Positive antinuclear antibodies or LE-cell test in association with characteristic clinical findings.	Occurs as isolated abnormality in slightly more than 10 per cent of cases. Effusion usually small, but may be moderate or even massive; bilateral in about 50 per cent. Usually clears without residua. Often associated with pericardial effusion. (*See* page 2723.)
Rheumatoid disease.	Serous exudate; tends to be turbid and greenish-yellow. Predominance of lymphocytes. Glucose concentration characteristically low, with failure to rise on IV glucose infusion (failure of glucose-transport mechanism).	Clinical or roentgenologic changes of rheumatoid arthritis. High titer of rheumatoid factor in serum highly suggestive but not conclusive. Biopsy of pleura showing typical rheumatoid granulation tissue.	Pleural fluid glucose abnormalities associated with one or more presumptive criteria.	Almost exclusively in men. Usually unilateral, on right slightly more often than on left. May antedate signs and symptoms of rheumatoid arthritis, but usually follows. Effusion often persists for several months. (*See* page 2725.)

NEOPLASTIC

Neoplasms arising within thorax: Lymphoma.	Usually serosanguineous exudate; may be chylous or chyliform.	Peripheral lymph node enlargement, hepatosplenomegaly, and so forth.	Finding of typical cells in pleural fluid or biopsy of pleura or lymph node.	This broad heading includes both Hodgkin's disease and non-Hodgkin's lymphoma. Approximately 30 per cent of cases have pleural effusion, but seldom without associated pulmonary or mediastinal node involvement. (*See* page 2729.)

Table continued on following page

Etiology	Character of the Fluid	Criteria for Presumptive Diagnosis	Criteria for Positive Diagnosis	Comments
NEOPLASTIC *(Continued)* Neoplasms arising outside the thorax:				
Metastatic carcinoma.	Serous exudate; varies in blood content from none to grossly hemorrhagic. Glucose content greater than 80 mg/100 ml is common but not diagnostic.	Identification of remote primary neoplasm.	Finding of characteristic tissue on needle biopsy or malignant cells in pleural fluid.	Most commonly from breast; also from pancreas, stomach, ovary, kidney. *(See page 2730.)*
Ovarian neoplasms (Meigs-Salmon syndrome).	Usually serous exudate; occasionally serosanguineous.	Pleural fluid negative for malignant cells; pelvic mass.	Presence of ovarian neoplasm with ascites; disappearance of effusion following oophorectomy.	Ovarian neoplasm may be fibroma, thecoma, cystadenoma, adenocarcinoma, granulosa-cell tumor; occasionally leiomyoma of uterus. *(See page 2737.)*
Carcinoma of the pancreas.	Serous exudate.	Pleural fluid negative for malignant cells; clinical signs of intra-abdominal neoplasia.	Disappearance of fluid following removal of primary.	Effusion may occur without direct involvement of thorax by primary; probably related to transport of fluid into thorax via diaphragmatic lymphatics. *(See page 2730.)*
Retroperitoneal lymphoma.	Serous exudate.	Pleural fluid negative for malignant cells; clinical signs of intra-abdominal neoplasia.	Disappearance of fluid following treatment of primary.	
Leukemia.	Serous exudate.	Disappearance of effusion following treatment of leukemia.	Demonstration of leukemic cells in peripheral blood.	Second in frequency only to mediastinal node enlargement. *(See page 2730.)*

THROMBOEMBOLIC

Pulmonary embolism.	Almost invariably serosanguineous.	History of sudden onset of pleural pain with or without peripheral thrombophlebitis. Rarely may observe relative diminution of peripheral vasculature roentgenologically.	Lung scan or pulmonary angiogram or both.	Frequency of effusion as sole manifestation of pulmonary embolism not precisely known, but probably very uncommon. (*See* page 2731.)

CARDIOVASCULAR

Cardiac decompensation.	Transudate.	Clinical signs of cardiac decompensation.	Disappearance of the fluid on treatment of the failure.	Frequently unilateral on the right, seldom on the left. (*See* page 2731.)

INHALATIONAL

Asbestosis.	Sterile, serous or blood-tinged exudate.	History of asbestos exposure.	Only following exclusion of other diagnostic possibilities, particularly tuberculosis and mesothelioma.	Diagnosis should be made with caution. Effusions frequently recurrent, usually bilateral, and often associated with chest pain. (*See* page 2727.)

TRAUMATIC

	Blood (hemothorax).	History.	Thoracentesis and history.	May originate from chest wall, diaphragm, mediastinum, or lung. (*See* page 2732.)
Closed-chest trauma.	Chyle (chylothorax).	History. Time lag between trauma and development of effusion.	Thoracentesis; lymphangiography.	Side of chylothorax depends on site of thoracic duct rupture. (*See* page 2735.)
	Contains ingested food (esophageal rupture).	History.	Thoracentesis; esophagogram.	Almost always left-sided. Generally due to surgical procedure. (*See* page 2732.)

Table continued on following page

TABLE 14
Pleural Effusion Unassociated With Other Roentgenographic Evidence of Disease in the Thorax *(Continued)*

Etiology	Character of the Fluid	Criteria for Presumptive Diagnosis	Criteria for Positive Diagnosis	Comments
TRAUMATIC *(Continued)* Following abdominal surgery.	Serous exudate.	History of recent abdominal surgery.	Unnecessary. Almost always self-limited.	Usually requires lateral decubitus roentgenograms for identification. Present in 49 per cent of patients in one series. *(See page 2736.)*
DRUG-INDUCED Bromcriptine. Methysergide. Dantrolene sodium. Nitrofurantoin.	Serous exudate.	History of specific drug therapy.	Resolution following withdrawal of the drug.	*(See Chapter 14, page 2417.)*
MISCELLANEOUS CAUSES Pancreatitis.	Usually serous exudate but may be serosanguineous. Pleural fluid amylase higher than serum amylase.	Clinical picture of acute abdomen.	Elevated level of pleural fluid anylase.	May occur in acute, chronic or relapsing pancreatitis. Majority of effusions are left-sided. *(See page 2736.)*
Nephrotic syndrome and other causes of diminished plasma osmotic pressure.	Transudate.	General edema.	Thoracentesis; biochemical assay of serum and urine.	Effusion commonly infrapulmonary. *(See page 2738.)*
Acute glomerulonephritis.	Transudate.	Usual findings of acute glomerulonephritis.	——	*(See page 2738.)*

104

Myxedema.	Serous exudate.	Studies of thyroid activity.	———	Effusion occurs more often in pericardium. (*See* page 2738.)
Cirrhosis with ascites.	Transudate.	Demonstration of cirrhosis and ascites. (N.B.: exclude carcinoma of liver.)	———	Ascitic fluid enters pleural space via diaphragmatic lymphatics (as in Meigs-Salmon syndrome). (*See* page 2738.)
Hydronephrosis and urinothorax.	Serous exudate.	Demonstration of hydronephrosis.	Disappearance of effusion following removal of urinary obstruction.	Mechanism not clear; possibly related to transport of fluid via diaphragmatic lymphatics. (*See* page 2737.)
Uremic pleuritis.	Serous exudate. Sometimes fibrinous.	Clinical findings of uremia.	———	May not be possible to distinguish from effusion associated with dialysis. (*See* page 2738.)
Dialysis.	Serous exudate, sometimes sanguineous as a result of anticoagulation.	History of peritoneal or hemodialysis.	———	May not be possible to distinguish from effusion associated with uremia itself. (*See* page 2737.)
Lymphedema.	High protein content.	Associated clinical findings of lymphedema elsewhere.	———	Results from hypoplasia of the lymphatic system. May be associated with Milroy's disease. (*See* page 2738.)

Table continued on following page

TABLE 14
Pleural Effusion Unassociated With Other Roentgenographic Evidence of Disease in the Thorax *(Continued)*

Etiology	Character of the Fluid	Criteria for Presumptive Diagnosis	Criteria for Positive Diagnosis	Comments
MISCELLANEOUS CAUSES *(Continued)*				
Familial recurring polyserositis.	Serofibrinous exudate.	Combination of symptoms and signs in specific racial groups.	———	Heredofamilial; limited to Armenians, Arabs, and Jews. Episodic acute attacks of abdominal and chest pain. Most episodes of pleurisy associated with arthritis and arthralgia. *(See* page 2739.)
Dressler's syndrome.	Serosanguineous exudate.	History of myocardial infarction or surgical procedure on the pericardium.	———	Syndrome can occur years after the causative episode. *(See* page 2739.)

TABLE 15

**Pleural Effusion Associated With Other
Roentgenographic Evidence of Disease in the Thorax**

This table includes all diseases in which unilateral or bilateral pleural effusion is associated with roentgenologic evidence of another abnormality in the thorax — local or general pulmonary disease, hilar or mediastinal lymph node enlargement, cardiomegaly, diaphragmatic abnormality, disease of the pleura, bony thorax, or chest wall, or any combination of these. This widely ranging list makes a long and rather cumbersome table; however, it seemed preferable to create a single, all-inclusive table than to subdivide diseases into separate categories according to the anatomic structures involved.

TABLE 15
Pleural Effusion Associated With Other Roentgenographic Evidence of Disease in the Thorax

Etiology	Character of the Fluid	Criteria for Presumptive Diagnosis	Criteria for Positive Diagnosis	Comments
INFECTIOUS				
Bacteria				
Klebsiella-Enterobacter-Serratia genera.	Purulent; predominant polymorphonuclear response.	Cavitating airspace pneumonia, often in upper lobes.	Culture of organism from sputum or pleural fluid.	Acute airspace pneumonia; cavitation frequent. Involved lobe may be expanded. (*See* page 2720.)
Francisella tularensis (tularemia).	Serous.	Combination of spherical or oval pulmonary densities with enlarged hilar nodes. History of animal exposure.	Rising serum agglutinin titers against *F. tularensis*. Isolation of the organism from sputum or pleural fluid.	Pleural effusion in 25 to 50 per cent of pneumonias. Hilar lymph node enlargement frequent. Pulmonary and pleural involvement much more frequent in typhoidal form (50 to 77 per cent) than in nontyphoidal (8 to 26 per cent). (*See* page 2721.)
Staphylococcus aureus.	Usually purulent but may be serous or serosanguineous.	In infants and children, pneumonia and empyema almost pathognomonic, particularly with abscess and pneumatocele formation.	Identification of organism by smear or culture from sputum or pleural fluid.	Rapidly progressive pneumonia — typically confluent segmental bronchopneumonia. Empyema more common in children (90 per cent) than in adults (50 per cent). (*See* page 2720.)
Streptococcus pneumoniae.	Serous.	Typical roentgen characteristics of acute airspace pneumonia.	Isolation of organism.	Demonstrable effusion very uncommon on standard roentgenograms in erect position. (*See* page 2720.)

Mycobacterium tuberculosis.	Serous or purulent.	Positive PPD reaction	Granulomas on pleural biopsy; acid-fast organisms on smear of sputum or pleural fluid. Culture of organism from sputum or pleural fluid.	Combined pleural effusion and roentgenographically demonstrable parenchymal disease an uncommon manifestation of either primary or postprimary tuberculosis. Effusion may occur as a manifestation of widely disseminated hematogenous disease or disease of the thoracic skeleton. (*See* page 2717.)
Yersinia pestis (the plague).	Serous.	Combination of confluent pneumonia, enlarged peripheral lymph nodes, and history of animal exposure.	Isolation of organism from sputum, blood, or aspirate of lymph node.	Pulmonary disease may simulate acute pulmonary edema. (*See* page 850.)
Streptococcus pyogenes.	Varies from serous effusion to frank pus.	———	Smear or culture of organism from pleural fluid (may be very difficult to identify).	Inhomogeneous or homogeneous segmental bronchopneumonia; abscess formation variable. In children, commonly preceded by viral disease, especially exanthems. (*See* page 2720.)

Table continued on following page

TABLE 15
Pleural Effusion Associated With Other Roentgenographic Evidence of Disease in the Thorax *(Continued)*

Etiology	Character of the Fluid	Criteria for Presumptive Diagnosis	Criteria for Positive Diagnosis	Comments
INFECTIOUS *(Continued)* **Bacteria** *(Continued)* *Pseudomonas aeruginosa.*				Homogeneous segmental bronchopneumonia. (*See* page 855.)
Escherichia coli.				Acute airspace pneumonia, commonly multilobar. (*See* page 849.)
Salmonella species.	Purulent.	Characteristically in patients with low resistance — e.g., chronic diseases, alcoholism.	Isolation of organism.	Segmental bronchopneumonia; abscess formation variable. Involvement of GI tract may not be obvious. (*See* page 850.)
Acinetobacter calcoaceticus.				Pneumonia, commonly with abscesses. Pyopneumothorax usually owing to bronchopleural fistula. (*See* page 868.)
Haemophilus influenzae.				Inhomogeneous segmental bronchopneumonia. In children, associated with acute upper respiratory tract symptoms. (*See* page 853.)

Anaerobic organisms.	Purulent	Characteristically in patients with low resistance — e.g., chronic diseases, alcoholism, and poor oral hygiene.	Isolation of organisms.	Segmental bronchopneumonia; incidence of infection higher than generally believed; organism requires anaerobic culture; may be intrapleural gas production. (*See* page 875.)
Actinomyces israelii (actinomycosis). *Nocardia* species.	Purulent.	Combination of cavitary pneumonia, pleural effusion (empyema), and chest wall involvement should strongly suggest these etiologies.	Isolation of organism from sputum, pleural fluid, or chest wall abscess.	Homogeneous nonsegmental airspace pneumonia almost invariable; abscess formation and chest wall involvement common, sometimes with rib destruction. Empyema necessitatis. (*See* pages 1022 and 1028.)
Fungi *Blastomyces dermatitidis.* *Cryptococcus neoformans.*	Serous exudate.	None.	Isolation of organism.	Effusion very uncommon in blastomycosis and rare in cryptococcosis. Associated with homogeneous nonsegmental airspace pneumonia; cavitation uncommon (15 per cent). Chest-wall involvement rare. (*See* pages 968 and 975.)
Aspergillus species.	Nonpurulent serous exudate.	None.	Isolation of organism.	Usually an opportunistic invader in postoperative empyema cavity; does not form pus. (*See* page 988.)

111

_ref id="1" />

Table continued on following page

TABLE 15
Pleural Effusion Associated With Other Roentgenographic Evidence of Disease in the Thorax *(Continued)*

Etiology	Character of the Fluid	Criteria for Presumptive Diagnosis	Criteria for Positive Diagnosis	Comments
INFECTIOUS *(Continued)* **Viruses**				
All viruses and *Mycoplasma pneumoniae.*	Serous exudate.	May be suggested by acute segmental pneumonia with combined interstitial and airspace elements. Clinical picture helpful.	Positive serologic tests. Isolation of organism.	Combined interstitial and airspace pneumonia (segmental). Effusion uncommon. (*See* page 1035.)
Parasites				
Entamoeba histolytica (amebiasis).	Usually serofibrinous but may become frankly purulent when secondarily infected. Occasionally fluid contains bile and necrotic liver tissue and then possesses characteristic "chocolate-sauce" appearance.	Combination of lower lobe consolidation, pleural effusion, and enlarged liver, especially in a patient with diarrhea.	Recovery of cysts or trophozoites from sputum, pleural fluid, or stool.	Elevation and fixation of right hemidiaphragm; homogeneous consolidation of right lower lobe, with or without abscess formation. Organisms infiltrate from liver abscess through diaphragm into pleura and lung. May form bronchohepatic fistula. (*See* page 1081.)
Paragonimus westermani.	Serous exudate.	Thin-walled cystic spaces in lower lobes in a patient from an endemic area.	Recovery of ova from sputum or feces.	Isolated nodular opacities, usually in lower lobes, commonly with cavitation. Metacercariae migrate from free peritoneal space through diaphragm into the pleura and lung. (*See* page 1109.)

Echinococcus granulosus (hydatid disease).	Cloudy serous fluid.	Commonly hydropneumothorax; floating scolices and daughter cysts producing "water lily" sign.	Positive Casoni skin test or complement fixation test. Recovery of hooklets from sputum or pleural fluid.	Pleural effusion develops as a result of rupture of a pulmonary hydatid cyst; a collapsed cystic space may be observed in the lungs; other solid hydatid cysts may be present. Rupture more commonly occurs into bronchus. (*See* page 1102.)
Extrathoracic infection Subphrenic abscess.	Serous exudate.	Elevated fixed hemidiaphragm with basal atelectasis and effusion (usually small).	Gas and fluid in subphrenic space.	Hemidiaphragm elevated and fixed; usually basal atelectasis, with or without pneumonia. (*See* page 2736.)
IMMUNOLOGIC Systemic lupus erythematosus.	Serous exudate.	Combination of bilateral pleural effusion, nonspecific cardiac enlargement, and basal atelectasis or pneumonia should suggest the diagnosis.	Positive antinuclear antibodies in association with characteristic clinical findings.	Pulmonary changes nonspecific – generally in form of basal "pneumonitis" or atelectasis; cardiac enlargement in 30 to 50 per cent of all cases, commonly due to pericardial effusion. Progressive loss of lung volume may be a characteristic. (*See* page 2723.)
Rheumatoid disease.	Exudate (*see* Table 14); low serum glucose values.	Pleuropulmonary disease in patients with rheumatoid arthritis.	High titer of rheumatoid factor in blood suggestive but not conclusive.	Diffuse reticulonodular pattern, predominantly basal in distribution. Pleural effusion most commonly an isolated finding; incidence of coexistent pleural effusion and pulmonary disease not clear but probably independent. (*See* page 2725.)

Table continued on following page

TABLE 15
Pleural Effusion Associated With Other Roentgenographic Evidence of Disease in the Thorax (Continued)

Etiology	Character of the Fluid	Criteria for Presumptive Diagnosis	Criteria for Positive Diagnosis	Comments
IMMUNOLOGIC (Continued)				
Wegener's granulomatosis.	Exudate.	Combination of pleural effusion and single or multiple pulmonary nodules (with or without cavitation), especially if associated with renal disease.	Biopsy of pulmonary or renal lesions.	Effusion was present in 6 of 11 cases in one series. (See page 1241.)
NEOPLASTIC				
Pulmonary carcinoma.	Serous exudate; may be sanguineous.	Obstructive pneumonitis with pleural effusion very strong presumptive evidence *per se.*	Recovery of cells from pleural fluid or sputum; positive pleural, bronchoscopic, or mediastinal node biopsy.	Commonly associated with obstructive pneumonitis. May or may not be associated with hilar or mediastinal node enlargement. Although the effusion may not contain cells, its presence is ominous. (See page 2729.)
Lymphoma.	Serosanguineous or chylous.	Combination of zones of consolidation (commonly separate from hilum) and pleural effusion, especially with enlargement of hilar and mediastinal nodes, constitutes strong presumptive evidence.	Biopsy of pleura, lung, or lymph node. Recovery of cells from pleural fluid.	Includes Hodgkin's disease and non-Hodgkin's lymphoma. Single or multiple areas of consolidated lung of varying size — may be massive; usually homogeneous. Hilar and mediastinal nodes also may be enlarged. Parenchymal involvement seldom if ever the presenting feature. (See page 2729.)

Metastatic carcinoma.	Serous or serosanguineous.	Combination of diffuse pulmonary densities and pleural effusion highly suggestive, particularly if heart size is normal; differentiation from bronchioloalveolar carcinoma may be difficult.	Identification of primary lesion; positive pleural biopsy or malignant cells in pleural fluid; cells occasionally identified in sputum.	Hematogenous: generally nodular. Lymphangitic: often predominantly linear but may have nodular component. Hilar and mediastinal nodes may be involved but this is seldom a prominent roentgenographic feature. (*See* page 2730.)
Mesothelioma.	Almost invariably bloody; hyaluronic acid levels may be elevated.	In local variety, peripherally situated mass usually having obtuse angles with chest wall. In diffuse type, history of exposure to asbestos. Volume of ipsilateral hemithorax may be reduced despite massive opacification.	Recovery of cells from pleural fluid. Positive pleural biopsy.	Effusion uncommon in local variety but almost invariable in diffuse malignant type. Either local or diffuse variety may be obscured by pleural fluid. (*See* page 2770.)
Bronchioloalveolar carcinoma.	Serous or serosanguineous.	High index of suspicion. Difficult to differentiate from metastatic neoplasm or widely disseminated lymphoma.	Malignant cells in pleural fluid or sputum. Biopsy.	Widely disseminated nodular densities of variable size, generally discrete but may be confluent in areas. Lymph nodes enlarged pathologically in 25 per cent of cases but may not be apparent roentgenologically. (*See* page 2729.)
Multiple myeloma.	Commonly serosanguineous.	Single or multiple soft-tissue masses arising from chest wall and protruding into thoracic space. Expansion of ribs almost pathognomonic.	Rib or chest wall biopsy; characteristic changes in bone marrow; electrophoretic pattern of serum proteins. Plasma cells may be numerous in pleural fluid.	Pleural effusion uncommon. Destructive lesions of one or more ribs with or without expansion. Soft-tissue masses commonly protrude into thorax. Also destructive lesions in shoulder girdle or thoracic spine. Lungs may be involved. (*See* page 2730.)

Table continued on following page

TABLE 15
Pleural Effusion Associated With Other Roentgenographic Evidence of Disease in the Thorax *(Continued)*

Etiology	Character of the Fluid	Criteria for Presumptive Diagnosis	Criteria for Positive Diagnosis	Comments
NEOPLASTIC *(Continued)* Primary neoplasms of chest wall.	Serosanguineous.	Combination of expanding lesion of chest wall and pleural effusion highly suggestive. May be indistinguishable from myeloma unless the latter is multiple.	Malignant cells in pleural fluid or biopsy.	Osteolytic, osteoblastic, or mixed neoplasms of ribs (or occasionally thoracic vertebrae) may extend into thoracic cavity. Primary mesenchymal neoplasms of intercostal spaces may act similarly. (*See* page 2955.)
Neoplastic involvement of pleura by direct invasion of a nonpulmonary carcinoma.	Serosanguineous.	In breast carcinoma, absence of breast shadow or history of mastectomy suggestive but not conclusive.	Typical cells in pleural fluid; pleural biopsy.	May occur occasionally from breast carcinoma, and rarely from liver or pancreas neoplasm. (*See* page 2730.)
Waldenström's macroglobulinemia.	Serous.	Diffuse reticulonodular pattern in the lungs of a patient with anemia, lymphocytic or plasmacytoid infiltration of the bone marrow, and monoclonal IgM gammopathy.	Lung biopsy. IgM gammopathy in blood and pleural fluid.	Effusion occurs in roughly 50 per cent of cases with lung involvement. (*See* page 2730.)
THROMBOEMBOLIC Pulmonary embolism and infarction.	Serosanguineous.	Any basal shadow associated with diaphragmatic elevation and pleural effusion should suggest the possibility. Clinical picture usually distinctive. Positive ventilation-perfusion scan highly suggestive.	Pulmonary angiogram.	Pulmonary changes vary from major segmental area of consolidation to line shadows of varying extent. Hemidiaphragm commonly elevated. Pleural effusion almost always small. (*See* page 2731.)

CARDIOVASCULAR

Cardiac decompensation.	Transudate.	Cardiac enlargement, usually general and "nonspecific." Clinical signs of cardiac decompensation.	Nature of the fluid on thoracentesis; its disappearance with treatment of cardiac decompensation.	Most commonly with failure of both sides of the heart. Frequently unilateral on the right, seldom on the left, but may be bilateral. (*See* page 2731.)
Constrictive pericarditis.	Transudate.	Signs of systemic venous hypertension.	Pericardial calcification with reduced amplitude of pulsation.	Effusion present in approximately 50 per cent of cases. (*See* page 2731.)
Obstruction of superior vena cava or azygos vein.	Transudate.	Clinical signs of superior vena cava syndrome.	Angiography or CT.	(*See* page 2879.)

INHALATIONAL

Asbestos-related disease.	Sterile, serous, or blood-tinged exudate.	History of asbestos exposure plus background of pulmonary asbestosis.	Only following exclusion of other diagnostic possibilities, particularly tuberculosis and mesothelioma.	Effusions frequently recurrent, usually bilateral and often associated with chest pain. Association with asbestosis is more common than pleural effusion alone. (*See* page 2727.)

TRAUMATIC

Open- or closed-chest trauma.	Blood (hemothorax). Chyle (chylothorax). Ingested food (esophageal rupture).	Associated findings should allow precise diagnosis in majority of cases.	Thoracentesis always diagnostic with positive history.	Wide variety of changes, including fractured ribs, pulmonary hemorrhage or hematoma, mediastinal hematoma, aortic aneurysm, pneumothorax, pneumomediastinum. (*See* page 2732.)

Table continued on following page

TABLE 15
Pleural Effusion Associated With Other Roentgenographic Evidence of Disease in the Thorax (Continued)

Etiology	Character of the Fluid	Criteria for Presumptive Diagnosis	Criteria for Positive Diagnosis	Comments
IDIOPATHIC Sarcoidosis.	Exudate containing a predominance of lymphocytes.	Association with biopsy-proved pulmonary sarcoidosis.	Identification of nonnecrotizing granulomas on pleural biopsy.	Invariably associated with pulmonary sarcoidosis, often of moderately advanced form. Incidence ranges from 0.7 to 7 per cent. (*See* page 2611.)
Lymphangioleiomyomatosis. Tuberous sclerosis.	Chylous.	Presence of numerous sclerotic lesions in the skeleton, renal angiomyolipomas, and intracranial calcifications in tuberous sclerosis.	Typical changes on lung biopsy. Diffuse reticulonodular pattern in a young woman in lymphangioleiomyomatosis.	Effusion can occur rarely in the absence of pulmonary disease and is rare in tuberous sclerosis. (*See* page 2673.)

118

TABLE 16

Hilar and Mediastinal Lymph Node Enlargement

This table includes all conditions producing lymph node enlargement within the thorax, either alone or in combination with other roentgenographic abnormalities. It is to be noted that a number of diseases are included in which node enlargement is a common manifestation in infants and children but uncommon in adults; since we have excluded much reference to pediatric diseases of the chest in the text, their inclusion here is a compromise to space limitation.

TABLE 16

Etiology	Symmetry	Node Groups Involved	Additional Findings	Comments
INFECTIOUS				
Bacteria				
Mycobacterium tuberculosis (primary).	Unilateral in 80 per cent of cases.	Approximately 60 per cent hilar and 40 per cent combined hilar and paratracheal.	Almost always associated with ipsilateral parenchymal disease.	Rarely the presentation may be bilateral, symmetric hilar node enlargement as sole manifestation. (*See* page 894.)
Francisella tularensis.	Unilateral.	Hilar.	Oval areas of parenchymal consolidation; pleural effusion common.	Ipsilateral hilar node enlargement in 25 to 50 per cent of pneumonic tularemia. (*See* page 870.)
Bordetella pertussis.	Unilateral.	Hilar.	Ipsilateral segmental pneumonia.	Pneumonia is the result of secondary infection in some cases. (*See* page 869.)
Bacillus anthracis.	Symmetric.	All.	Occasionally patchy nonsegmental opacities throughout lungs due to pulmonary hemorrhage; pleural effusion is common.	Node enlargement due to hemorrhage and edema; extension of inflammatory reaction into adjacent mediastinal tissues may obscure typical nodal configuration. (*See* page 842.)
Yersinia pestis (the plague).	Symmetric.	Hilar and paratracheal.	——	Rarely, roentgenographic changes may be restricted to node enlargement, without associated pulmonary manifestations. (*See* page 850.)

Fungi

Histoplasma capsulatum.	May be unilateral or bilateral.	Hilar or paratracheal or both.	Enlarged nodes may obstruct airways through extrinsic pressure, resulting in obstructive pneumonitis and atelectasis.	Node enlargement is usually associated with parenchymal disease but may occur without, particularly in children. (*See* page 949.)
Coccidioides immitis.	Unilateral or bilateral.	Hilar or paratracheal or both.	Node enlargement may occur with or without associated parenchymal disease.	Involvement of paratracheal lymph nodes should raise suspicion of imminent dissemination. (*See* page 957.)
Sporothrix schenkii.	Unilateral.	Hilar.	Associated with parenchymal disease in some cases.	A rare form of mycotic infection. (*See* page 1019.)

Mycoplasma and viruses

Mycoplasma pneumoniae.	Unilateral or bilateral.	Hilar.	Always with segmental inhomogeneous or homogeneous pneumonia.	Lymph node enlargement is rare in adults but common in children. (*See* page 1036.)
Rubeola.	Bilateral.	Hilar.	Diffuse interstitial pattern throughout the lungs.	This pattern results from infection with rubeola virus itself and not from secondary infection. (*See* page 1050.)
ECHO virus.	Bilateral.	Hilar.	Accompanied by increase in bronchovascular markings.	Lymph node enlargement rare in adults and pneumonia extremely rare in infants. (*See* page 1056.)
Varicella-zoster.	Bilateral.	Hilar.	Diffuse airspace pneumonia may mask hilar node enlargement.	(*See* page 1062.)
Chlamydia psittaci (ornithosis).	Unilateral or bilateral.	Hilar.	Parenchymal involvement may be homogeneous consolidation or a diffuse reticular pattern.	Hilar node enlargement has not been reported as sole manifestation of the disease. (*See* page 1074.)

Table continued on following page

TABLE 16
Hilar and Mediastinal Lymph Node Enlargement *(Continued)*

Etiology	Symmetry	Node Groups Involved	Additional Findings	Comments
INFECTIOUS *(Continued)* **Mycoplasma and viruses** *(Continued)*				
Epstein-Barr mononucleosis.	Bilateral symmetric.	Predominantly hilar.	Splenomegaly.	Rarely associated with roentgenographic changes in the lungs. (*See* page 1071.)
Parasites Tropical eosinophilia.	Bilateral.	Hilar.	A widespread micronodular pattern throughout the lungs.	Diffuse parenchymal disease is usually not accompanied by node enlargement. (*See* page 1097.)
IMMUNOLOGIC Extrinsic allergic alveolitis.	Symmetric.	Bronchopulmonary.	Diffuse reticulonodular (sometimes acinar) pattern invariably associated.	Hilar node enlargement fairly common in mushroom-workers' lung but rare in other varieties. (*See* page 1273.)
NEOPLASTIC Pulmonary carcinoma.	Unilateral almost invariably.	Hilar nodes usually; paratracheal and posterior mediastinal nodes in some cases.	Involvement of the bifurcation or posterior mediastinal groups of nodes may displace the barium-filled esophagus.	Enlargement of mediastinal lymph nodes may be the sole abnormality roentgenographically and almost always indicates spread from a small cell carcinoma. (*See* page 1415.)

Hodgkin's disease.	Typically bilateral but asymmetric; unilateral node enlargement is very unusual.	Paratracheal and bifurcation group involved as often as or more often than bronchopulmonary group. Involvement of anterior mediastinal and retrosternal nodes frequent.	Pulmonary involvement occurs in less than 30 per cent of patients and is almost invariably associated with mediastinal node enlargement. Pleural effusion in approximately 30 per cent of cases, usually in association with other intrathoracic manifestations. The sternum may be destroyed by direct extension from retrosternal nodes.	Intrathoracic involvement occurs in 90 per cent of patients at some stage of the disease, most commonly in the form of mediastinal lymph node enlargement; the latter is seen on the initial chest roentgenogram in approximately 50 per cent of patients. (*See* page 1507.)
Non-Hodgkin's lymphoma.	Bilateral but asymmetric.	Similar to Hodgkin's disease.	Sometimes associated with pleuropulmonary involvement.	The most common intrathoracic manifestation of the disease; however, large cell lymphoma tends to be manifested by parenchymal consolidation without associated node enlargement. (*See* page 1535.)
Leukemia.	Usually symmetric.	Mediastinal and hilar.	Both pleural effusion and parenchymal involvement may be associated.	The most common roentgenographic manifestation of leukemia within the thorax (25 per cent of patients). A much more common manifestation of lymphocytic than of myelocytic leukemia. (*See* page 1554.)
Lymphangitic carcinomatosis.	Unilateral or bilateral.	Hilar or mediastinal or both.	Usually associated with a diffuse reticular or reticulonodular pattern throughout the lungs, predominantly basal in distribution.	Septal (Kerley B) lines are frequently present. (*See* page 1632.)
Bronchioloalveolar carcinoma.	Unilateral or bilateral.	Hilar or mediastinal or both.	Node enlargement may occur in association with either local or diffuse pulmonary disease.	A rare finding in this neoplasm. (*See* page 1414.)

123

Table continued on following page

TABLE 16
Hilar and Mediastinal Lymph Node Enlargement *(Continued)*

Etiology	Symmetry	Node Groups Involved	Additional Findings	Comments
NEOPLASTIC *(Continued)* Angioimmunoblastic lymphadenopathy.	Bilateral but asymmetric.	Similar to Hodgkin's disease.	The lungs are occasionally affected in a pattern similar to that in Hodgkin's disease.	A hyperimmune disorder, most probably of B lymphocytes. Lymph node enlargement predominates and is identical to that of Hodgkin's disease. (*See* page 1570.)
INHALATIONAL Silicosis.	Symmetric.	Predominantly hilar.	Diffuse nodular or reticulonodular disease throughout both lungs. Pleural thickening in late stages. Eggshell calcification of lymph nodes occurs in approximately 5 per cent of cases and may also be observed in lymph nodes in the anterior and posterior mediastinum, the thoracic wall, and occasionally the retroperitoneal and intraperitoneal nodes.	Enlargement of hilar nodes may occur without roentgenographic evidence of pulmonary disease, although this is a rare presenting picture. (*See* page 2289.)
Chronic berylliosis.	Symmetric.	Hilar.	Diffuse micronodular pattern invariably associated.	Hilar node enlargement occurs in a minority of cases. (*See* page 2363.)

IDIOPATHIC				
Sarcoidosis.	Almost invariably symmetric, unilateral node enlargement occurring in 1 to 3 per cent of cases only. The outer borders of the enlarged hila are usually lobulated.	Paratracheal, tracheobronchial, and bronchopulmonary groups. Paratracheal enlargement seldom if ever occurs without concomitant enlargement of hilar nodes.	75 to 90 per cent of patients with sarcoid show mediastinal and hilar lymph node enlargement and approximately 40 per cent of these show diffuse parenchymal disease as well.	75 per cent of patients with hilar lymph node enlargement show complete resolution of the enlarged nodes. Symmetric appearance, lack of involvement of retrosternal nodes, and diminution of lymph node size with onset of diffuse lung disease aid in differentiating sarcoidosis from lymphoma and tuberculosis. (*See* page 2611.)
Histiocytosis X (eosinophilic granuloma).	Symmetric.	Hilar and mediastinal.	Early diffuse micronodular pattern which may become coarse in later stages.	Intrathoracic lymph node enlargement is rarely a manifestation of this disease. (*See* page 2682.)
Idiopathic pulmonary hemorrhage.	Symmetric.	Hilar.	Diffuse alveolar and interstitial disease.	Predominantly in acute stage. (*See* page 1183.)
AIRWAYS				
Cystic fibrosis.	Unilateral or bilateral.	Hilar.	Diffuse increase in markings with hyperinflation and areas of atelectasis and bronchiectasis.	Hilar node enlargement is an uncommon finding in this disease. (*See* page 2213.)
METABOLIC				
Bronchopulmonary amyloidosis.	Symmetric.	Hilar and mediastinal.	Enlarged nodes may be densely calcified.	Usually associated with diffuse pulmonary involvement. (*See* page 2578.)

TABLE 17

Mediastinal Widening

The conditions listed in this table include all those responsible for increase in the width or mass of the mediastinum. Of necessity, there is considerable overlap of diseases in Tables 16 and 17; since enlargement of lymph nodes causes mediastinal widening, it is clear that all diseases listed in Table 16 could be included in this category. However, in Table 17, emphasis is placed on those diseases that cause widening of the mediastinal silhouette in which contour does *not* suggest node enlargement.

The headings in this table include *anatomic location* of the various disease processes within the mediastinal compartments: the designation + + + indicates that the process is almost invariably within that compartment, + + that it predominates in that compartment, and + that it sometimes is located in that compartment. Thus, those diseases indicated by a single + in all compartments show no definite anatomic predilection. Where possible, the order in which the diseases are listed has been arranged to comply with predominant anatomic location; thus, under *Neoplastic,* tumors that tend to occupy the anterior compartment are listed first, the middle compartment second, and the posterior compartment last.

No attempt has been made to include diseases of the heart, since such clearly is outside the scope of this book. Similarly, abnormalities of mediastinal contour that relate directly or indirectly to cardiac anomalies have been excluded (e.g., the "snowman" configuration of anomalous pulmonary venous return).

TABLE 17
Mediastinal Widening

| Etiology | Location | | | Contour | Additional Findings | Comments |
	Anterior	Middle	Posterior			
DEVELOPMENTAL						
Bronchial cyst.	+	+ +	+ +	Round or oval, well defined. Contour may be affected by contact with more solid structures.	May compress tracheobronchial tree or esophagus. Calcification rare (however, *see* Figure 5–10, page 718.)	Cyst may be multilocular. Seldom communicates with tracheobronchial tree. May look like a solid mass on CT because of high attenuation of contents. (*See* page 714.)
Mesothelial cyst (pericardial and pleuropericardial cysts).	+	+ +		Usually round, oval, or "tear-drop" in appearance, with smooth margin.	Variation in shape of cyst may occur on changing position of patient.	Almost always do not cause symptoms. (*See* page 2867.)
Diverticula of the pharynx or esophagus.			+ + +	Cyst-like structure in superior (pharyngeal) or inferior (esophageal) regions.	Invariably communicate with pharynx or esophagus. May displace contiguous esophagus.	Aspiration pneumonia may develop from pharyngeal (Zenker's) diverticulum. (*See* page 2903.)
Gastroenteric (neurenteric) cyst.			+ + +	Oval or lobulated, sharply defined, homogeneous.	Spinal anomalies in many cases. Rarely air is found in cyst.	Often discovered in infancy. May reach large size, and may be unilateral or bilateral. (*See* page 2902.)
Meningocele and meningomyelocele.			+ + +	Sharply circumscribed, solitary or multiple, unilateral or bilateral.	Frequently spine and rib deformities. No calcification.	Usually communicate with spinal subarachnoid space. (*See* page 2901.)

INFECTIOUS

			Character	Additional Findings	Comments
Chronic sclerosing mediastinitis.	+	+	+	Lobulated, usually in right paramediastinal area.	May show calcification. Compression of SVC or other vessel or major airway in some cases.	The cause of approximately 10 per cent of mediastinal widening. (*See* page 2796.)
Acute mediastinitis.	+	+	+	Symmetric widening due to diffuse involvement or localized due to abscess formation.	May be air in mediastinum.	Most cases due to esophageal rupture. (*See* page 2796.)
Anthrax.	+	+		Symmetric widening resulting from hemorrhagic edema of lymph nodes.	Patchy nonsegmental opacities may be present in lungs, owing to hemorrhagic edema. Pleural effusion common.	Disease commonest in sorters and combers in the wool industry. Organism (*B. anthracis*) is extremely virulent. (*See* page 842.)
Suppurative spondylitis.			+ + +	Widening of lower mediastinum with fusiform mass.	Erosion or destruction of vertebrae at level of paravertebral mass.	(*See* page 2908.)

NEOPLASTIC
Tumors and tumor-like conditions of the thymus:

				Character	Additional Findings	Comments
Thymic hyperplasia.	+ + +				Smooth or lobulated.	None.	Defined as an increase in the size of the gland associated with an intact gross architecture and normal histologic appearance. (*See* page 2815.)

Table continued on following page

TABLE 17
Mediastinal Widening *(Continued)*

Etiology	Location			Contour	Additional Findings	Comments
	Anterior	Middle	Posterior			
NEOPLASTIC *(Continued)*						
Thymolipoma.	+ + +			Smooth or lobulated.	None.	These tumors can grow very large, and because of their fat content and soft pliable consistency tend to slump toward the diaphragm, leaving the upper mediastinum relatively clear. (*See* page 2818.)
Thymic cysts.	+ + +			Smooth.	None.	Cystic nature should be readily apparent on CT. (*See* page 2820.)
Thymoma.	+ + +			Smooth or lobulated; well defined.	Contains calcium in some cases.	Close relationship to myasthenia gravis. CT is the examination of choice. (*See* page 2820.)
Thymic neuroendocrine neoplasms.	+ + +			Lobulated.	Contain calcium in some cases.	Derived from neuroendocrine cells; the most common histologic type is carcinoid tumor. (*See* page 2831.)
Thymic carcinoma.	+ + +			Irregular, poorly defined.	Invasion of adjacent structures common at the time of diagnosis.	Bulky masses ranging from 5 to 15 cm in diameter. Prognosis poor. (*See* page 2834.)

Thymic lymphoma.	+++			Smooth or lobulated.	Mediastinal lymph node enlargement in some cases.	Hodgkin's disease and lymphoblastic lymphoma most common types. (*See* page 2835.)

Germ cell neoplasms:
  Teratoma.
  Seminoma.
  Choriocarcinoma.
  Endodermal sinus tumor.
		+++	+	Smooth or lobulated, oval or round. May protrude to either side or bilaterally.	Calcification, bone, teeth, or fat may be identified in teratomas.	CT or MRI is the examination of choice. (*See* page 2835.)

Thyroid tumors.	++		+	Smooth or lobulated.	Anterior tumors displace the trachea posteriorly and laterally; posterior tumors displace trachea anteriorly and esophagus posteriorly. Calcification fairly common.	Typically a nodular goiter. Radioactive isotopic studies are usually diagnostic although CT may be required. (*See* page 2844.)
Parathyroid tumors.	+++			Smooth or lobulated.	Evidence of hyperparathyroidism in the thoracic skeleton. Mass may displace esophagus.	Arteriography or CT may reveal smaller lesions. Hypercalcemia and hypophosphatemia. (*See* page 2846.)
Soft-tissue tumors and tumor-like conditions: Lipomatosis.	++	+	+	Smooth and symmetric; sometimes lobulated.	Enlargement of pleuropericardial fat pads.	Usually associated with Cushing's syndrome or long-term corticosteroid therapy, occasionally with simple obesity. If necessary, CT diagnostic. (*See* page 2848.)

Table continued on following page

TABLE 17
Mediastinal Widening *(Continued)*

Etiology	Location			Contour	Additional Findings	Comments
	Anterior	Middle	Posterior			
NEOPLASTIC *(Continued)*						
Lipoma. Liposarcoma. Hemangioma. Angiosarcoma. Hemangiopericytoma. Lymphangioma. Leiomyoma. Leiomyosarcoma. Fibroma. Fibrosarcoma.	+ +	+	+	Commonly smooth and well defined.	Variable.	Each of these tumors can occur in any mediastimal compartment but are usually located anteriorly. (*See* pages 2846 to 2858.)
Lymphoma and leukemia.	+ +	+ + +		Symmetrically widened mediastinum or solitary or multiple lobulated masses.	Pulmonary consolidation and pleural effusion in some cases.	Most common mediastinal "mass." (*See* page 2858.)
Metastatic lymph node enlargement.	+	+ + +	+	Commonly unilateral with pulmonary carcinoma. Predominant involvement may occur in paratracheal or hilar groups.	Phrenic nerve involvement may result in diaphragmatic paralysis.	Primary usually pulmonary carcinoma. May originate from GI tract, breast, kidney, and so forth. (*See* page 1415.)

132

Giant lymph node hyperplasia.	+	+ + +	+	Usually solitary and sharply circumscribed.	No calcification.	In anterior mediastinum a multilobulated appearance may suggest thymic or teratoid tumors. (*See* page 2861.)
Tumors and tumor-like conditions of neural tissue:						
Aorticopulmonary paraganglioma (chemodectoma).		+ + +		Smooth or lobulated.	None.	A neoplasm of the extra-adrenal paraganglionic system, arising from aorticopulmonary paraganglia. (*See* page 2866.)
Aorticosympathetic (paravertebral) paraganglioma.			+ + +	Smooth or lobulated.	None.	Arises from segmental ganglia of the sympathetic chain in the posterior mediastinum. (*See* page 2901.)
Tumors of peripheral nerves (neurofibroma, neurilemoma, neurogenic sarcoma). Tumors of sympathetic ganglia (ganglioneuroma, ganglioneuroblastoma, neuroblastoma).			+ + +	Round or oval, well defined. Rarely dumbbell-shaped.	Majority are paravertebral in location, usually unilateral. Rib or vertebral erosion variable. Rarely calcification in tumor.	CT, with or without myelography, usually required for diagnosis. (*See* page 2898.)

Table continued on following page

TABLE 17
Mediastinal Widening (Continued)

Etiology	Location			Contour	Additional Findings	Comments
	Anterior	Middle	Posterior			
NEOPLASTIC (Continued)						
Esophageal neoplasms.			+ + +	Smooth, rounded margin; usually unilateral.	Smooth compression of esophageal lumen on barium swallow.	Usually carcinoma or leiomyoma. (See page 2903.)
Bone and cartilage neoplasms.	+		+ + +	Rounded, paravertebral mass.	Destruction of affected bone, often associated with soft tissue mass protruding into and compressing lung.	(See page 2908.)
CARDIOVASCULAR						
Aortic aneurysm.	+	+	+	Fusiform or saccular.	Erosion of bony thoracic cage where pulsatile aneurysm is contiguous. Calcification may be present in wall.	Aortography or CT may be needed for definitive diagnosis. (See page 2885.)
Buckling or aneurysm of the innominate artery.		+ + +		Smooth, lateral bulging, convex laterally from level of aortic arch upwards.	Tortuous thoracic aorta due to atherosclerosis may also be noted.	Angiography or CT may be required for definitive diagnosis but is seldom indicated. (See page 2888.)
Superior vena caval dilatation.		+ + +		Smooth, extending from hilum along right paramediastinal border.	Signs of etiology — e.g., cardiac dilatation, mediastinal mass, and so forth.	Secondary to central pressure rise or to compression and obstruction. (See page 2879.)

Condition				Radiologic Findings	Associated Findings	Comments
Azygos and hemiazygos dilatation.		+	+ +	Smooth, round or oval mass at tracheobronchial angle.	Change in size with Valsalva and Mueller procedures and with change in body position.	Azygography or CT may be required for definitive diagnosis. (*See* page 2879.)
Dilatation of pulmonary artery.		+ + +		Smooth.	Stenotic pulmonary valve or peripheral vascular attenuation in secondary types.	Angiography or CT may be required to differentiate this from mediastinal tumors. (*See* page 2869.)
Aortic vascular ring.		+	+	A vessel situated between trachea and esophagus.	Compression of esophagus or trachea.	Usually detected in first year of life. (*See* page 731.)

TRAUMATIC

Condition				Radiologic Findings	Associated Findings	Comments
Pneumomediastinum.	+	+	+	Smooth; unilateral or bilateral.	Unilateral or bilateral pneumothorax. Subcutaneous and interstitial emphysema.	Much more commonly spontaneous. Readily diagnosed by presence of mediastinal air. (*See* page 2498.)
Mediastinal hemorrhage or hematoma.	+	+	+	May be local or diffuse, commonly in upper mediastinum.	Rarely SVC compression.	History of trauma (including surgery) or dissecting aneurysm. (*See* page 2499.)
Fracture of vertebra with hematoma.			+ + +	Smooth paravertebral swelling, usually bilateral.	Vertebral and rib fractures.	(*See* page 2908.)

Table continued on following page

TABLE 17
Mediastinal Widening *(Continued)*

Etiology	Location			Contour	Additional Findings	Comments
	Anterior	Middle	Posterior			
MISCELLANEOUS CAUSES						
Herniation through foramen of Morgagni.	+ + +			Round or oval; usually to right of pericardium.	If completely radiopaque, CT may differentiate this from epicardial fat or pericardial cyst.	Often in asymptomatic individuals. Examination of the colon may be diagnostic. (*See* page 2867.)
Esophageal hiatus hernia.			+ + +	Retrocardiac mass of variable size containing air and fluid; usually smooth.	May contain several fluid levels; rarely completely opaque. Barium usually outlines contents.	Contains stomach, rarely bowel, omentum, liver, or spleen. (*See* page 2906.)
Herniation through foramen of Bochdalek.			+ + +	Round or oval retrocardiac density. Unilateral and rarely bilateral.	———	Occasionally contains bowel loops, more often omentum or solid abdominal viscera. (*See* page 2908.)
Megaesophagus.			+ + +	Broad vertical opacity on the right side of the mediastinum.	Air in lumen with fluid level at varying distance from diaphragm.	Usually the result of progressive systemic sclerosis or achalasia. (*See* page 2906.)
Extramedullary hematopoiesis.			+ + +	Smooth or lobulated, usually bilateral.	Spleen may be enlarged.	Anemia and hepatosplenomegaly. (*See* page 2908.)

INDEX